eHealth—
A Global Perspective

Executive Editors and Contributing Authors

ALAN R. SHARK, D.P.A. and

SYLVIANE TOPORKOFF, PH.D.

PUBLIC TECHNOLOGY INSTITUTE AND ITEMS INTERNATIONAL

WASHINGTON, D.C.

Library of Congress Cataloging-Publication-Data
Toporkoff, Sylviane; Shark, Alan
eHealth—A Global Perspective
p. cm.
ISBN1451540299
EAN-13 9781451540291

Information technology-Management. 2. Health IT. I.Title

Contents

Preface

With billions of dollars being spent every year by governments around the world, the field of eHealth provides great hope in providing citizens with access to health information as never before, to streamline the very process of health-care delivery through better use of cutting-edge technology and to reduce costs through the efficiencies of technology applications.

During the past few Global Forum annual meetings, many discussions emerged regarding the dramatic progress in eHealth applications worldwide. The authors felt that the next book in the Global Perspective series should be on this very topic. We believe this is a topic that could not be more timely. This book contains an enlightened collection of information written by 24 practitioners and researchers around the globe. Many more wanted to contribute to this book but were unable to break away from the daily pressures to be able to find the time to write and share. Perhaps we can include them in the next edition. This book is not designed to be a how-to manual; instead, it was designed to offer insights as to the issues of the day and how various governments, institutions, and businesses are developing creative solutions utilizing the latest in technology.

We recognize the fact that some parts of this book could easily become shared information before the print ink even dries due to the rapidly changing nature of innovation and changes. Toward that end, we hope to be able to update this book on a periodic basis, and perhaps one of these days, we will offer an e-reader edition, too.

Many wonderful and talented people must be recognized for their direct and indirect involvement in this book. This, of course, begins with having the support and active engagement of two dozen remarkable author/contributors. Without their hard work and dedication, this book would not be possible, for they represent its soul and content.

At Items International, we wish to recognize Baila Sow for his help in collecting the information and Sébastien Lévy for his support of the overall publishing project. At PTI, and on the production side, many thanks go to Lindsay Isaacs, who served as the project's copy editor. Lindsay's job was quite a challenge in not only checking for common editorial edits, she had the daunting task of converting dozens of different international versions of Word into one cohesive document. We are also forever grateful to Sally Hoffmaster for her work as graphic designer for the cover and page layout of the entire manuscript.

Finally, we encourage you, the reader, to share your thoughts about this book and to consider contributing for a revised edition in the not-too-distant future.

Chapter 1

Health IT Trends and Opportunities in the United States and Europe

Dr. Alan R. Shark, D.P.A., and
Dr. Sylviane Toporkoff, Ph.D.

The United States

Health Care Information Technology in the U.S. has quickly moved from a rather obscure subject to one of great interest with serious economic and political implications. Some believe the main driver for healthcare reform in the U.S. is driven more by the alarming concern over escalating costs than the concern for providing improved coverage to its citizens. The United States is the only industrialized nation where health care benefits are mostly obtained through one's employment. In most instances, part-time or temporary workers do not receive any healthcare benefits, and if they do, they are minimal. For those who are unemployed or underemployed, the citizen must pay for his or her own healthcare policy or simply go without coverage. It is estimated that at least 30 million Americans (not counting illegal aliens) remain without any form of health coverage. To be fair, U.S. citizens are eligible for modest coverage through Medicaid and Medicare programs when they turn 65.

Health information technology (health IT) in the U.S. involves the exchange of health information in an electronic environment. Widespread use of health IT within the health care industry is designed to:

1. Improve the quality of health care
2. Prevent medical errors
3. Reduce health care costs
4. Eliminate duplicative services
5. Increase administrative efficiencies
6. Decrease paperwork
7. Expand access to affordable health care
8. Increase the speed and flow of medical payments to patients and providers

9. Promote greater statistical record gathering regarding costs, trends and practices

10. Provide privacy rights to patients and their families

11. Provide redress for violations

12. Provide standards for greater seamless interoperability

13. Enhance decision support through geographic information systems

Another characteristic of the U.S. healthcare system is that it is largely regulated at the state level and not at the federal level. Each state has its own insurance regulations, making it difficult and expensive for any national type of private company to operate in all 50 states. In one of the most sweeping changes in U.S. health care, the U.S. Congress enacted the Health Insurance Portability and Accountability Act (HIPAA) in 1996 that was designed to improve the efficiency and effectiveness of the nation's health care system by encouraging the widespread use of electronic data exchange as well as the privacy of one's health care records.

The U.S. spends $2.5 trillion dollars a year for healthcare—more than twice that of any other developed country in the world. Adding to the financial burden, 64% of Americans are either overweight or obese, and that number is expected to climb to 75% by the year 2015 with 41% considered obese. Another troubling statistic is the U.S. currently ranks 50th out of 244 nations in life expectancy, with an average life span of 78.1 years. When it comes to infant mortality, the U.S. ranks 30th in the world.

The healthcare debate currently going on in the U.S. has become a polarizing issue and has pitted various public and political interest groups against one another. But the health IT debate is not only about reducing costs and increasing coverage for those un-served or underserved, it is also about cutting into waste and fraud. One figure widely used by law enforcement officials suggests a staggering $60 billion a year is stolen from Medicaid programs, the national entitlement program, which funds medical treatment, equipment and prescriptions for 45 million seniors and the disabled. Even with a new comprehensive law, this debate will rage on for years to come, with many fearing a federal plan as being too costly and intrusive.

Regardless of what type of healthcare reform is ultimately decided, there is one major category where everyone agrees: the need to cut waste and duplication. This is one reason why health IT has remained on the forefront of planning, as technology, when properly applied, can reduce waste and duplication, and much more. Health IT alone will not be the sole solution in reducing costs, but it's a reasonable place to start.

Health IT is far more complex than simply focusing on patients' records. The operational term covers patients' rights for confidentiality as well as records transportability—that need to travel between patient, healthcare provider, insurance company, and perhaps government agencies at various levels. Health IT also refers to health information services found online on the Internet, distance learning of IT practices, telemedicine, and remote health monitoring devices. Health IT can also describe biosensors, which can help keep physicians up-to-date on the conditions of their chronically ill elderly patients, thus supporting increased life expectancy.

When it comes to savings, some experts estimate a savings of over $30 billion per year simply by moving away from a paper-based system to paperless online systems. Today, 90% of all medical claims are processed through the mail, with payments being mailed to the patient. Some estimate that $11 billion a year could be saved by simply depositing payments electronically into a patient's account. Today, the federal government is both encouraging and mandating electronic records and claims when filing Medicare claims.

The Health Insurance Portability and Accountability Act (HIPAA) was initially designed to help protect citizens medical records and to provide certain protections when a worker changes or loses a job. Lately more attention is focusing on another key component of HIPAA that requires the establishment of national standards for electronic healthcare transactions. The act has been expanded to include new and expanded protections and attempts to balance the needs of the patient as well as the need for the disclosure of personal health information needed for patient care and other important purposes.

Depending on whether one is a patient or a health care provider, the HIPAA regulatory framework is complex with stiff penalties for abuses or violations. This often leads to the common practice of requesting the patient, and perhaps their family, to sign a waiver as a condition of service.

HIPAA provides rights and protections for patients to have the ability to correct any errors in their medical records. It also establishes regulations for the use of Protected Health Information (PHI), which covers both medical records and payment history. Recognizing the need for even greater specificity in a growing technical environment, a new initiative called HIPAA 5010 is the federal government's response to issues posed by the first set of HIPAA standards. The healthcare industry has asked for more than 500 changes to the current HIPAA standards to support new business requirements and/or correct old problems. HIPAA 5010 addresses these issues and attempts to bring more value to the healthcare community with the aim of significantly eliminating many of the barriers to broader adoption regarding electronic records, reducing or eliminating the need for paper processing and telephone calls, and speeding up the process of payments for services. The new standards are supposed to take effect January 2012.

Health IT in a broad sense is rapidly growing in many other applications that go far beyond patient record privacy and paperless systems. With the dramatic growth of broadband adoption and Internet connectivity, both fixed and wireless health IT applications are spurning innovation in information, training, monitoring, and diagnostics. For example, the iPhone has added a "Medical" Category, offering thousands of medical applications, including information services and interactive activities. This new category is in addition to its already popular "Healthcare and Fitness Category." Diabetes monitoring devices can be wirelessly joined to one's smart phone as well as hundreds of wellness and prevention applications.

Health IT in its expanded definition covers telemedicine, e-learning and remote healthcare through broadband connectivity. The private sector, while watchful of Federal regulations, has developed applications for patient health records, which empower citizens to manage their own records and information online. A personal health record permits one to securely gather, store, manage and share a person's own and/or family's health information when they want it, where they want it, and with whom they choose. The advantages of why someone would want to create a personal health record are:

- ♦ To easily gather, store and manage lifelong personal health information
- ♦ To share relevant information with authorized care providers
- ♦ To maximize your health benefits

The private sector in the U.S. has decided to initiate Health IT applications on their own without waiting for the federal government to act and set national standards. Companies in the U.S. that offer personal medical records number in the hundreds, with better-known names such as WebMD, Microsoft with their Health Vault service, and Google Health, a collaboration between Google and IBM.

Health providers, like Kaiser Permanente, as well as hundreds of other healthcare providers offer innovative online portals—usually in more than one language and some offer mobile applications—that might include the ability to:

- ♦ E-mail a doctor
- ♦ Obtain test results
- ♦ Schedule appointments
- ♦ Refill prescriptions

- ◆ Review past visits
- ◆ Download and/or complete medical forms online
- ◆ Obtain specialist referrals

Most, if not all, of the above categories replace what has traditionally been transacted through the inefficiencies of telephone and mail transactions. The private sector is well aware of the advantages of automating patient care wherever it can to reduce time, waste, data entry, speed up administrative processes, speed up payments, and promote online services as a marketing tool to help sign up more customers.

Innovation in the U.S. is gaining where its baby-boomer citizens are aging and becoming more health conscious. At the same time, a younger generation that is highly computer- and wireless device literate are demanding more by way of online services and mobile applications. With the ever-expanding utility of social networking sites—such as Twitter, Facebook, YouTube, WebMD, to name a few—citizens have greater access to health information as never before. Governments around the world are not only taking note of this trend they are offering sites of their own, such as the Center for Disease Control, the World Health Organization, and the Departments of Health & Human Services all with special sub-sites for information and information interactivity, such as subscribing to RSS feeds, following on Twitter-type sites, and signing up to be part of other social networks.

ESRI is the U.S.-based company that is recognized as one of the world leaders in GIS (geographic information systems) modeling and mapping systems. They offer many solutions for policy-makers, administrators and researchers to track healthcare spending, analyze trends, as well as track and identify possible epidemic outbreaks by block, city, county or region. Afterall, GIS systems are based on sophisticated multi-level databases which, when integrated with GIS systems, provide critical real-time visual planning tools and alerts.

The U.S. experience with Health IT has evolved through expanded definitions and innovative applications to better serve citizens utilizing the latest technology, and as technology morphs into new breakthroughs, so, too, will health IT. The private sector, out of necessity, has taken a lead in developing innovative health IT solutions, and the federal government has played a key leadership role in protecting citizens and the exchange of records and information through the better use of technology.

Europe

The benefits of eHealth for a safer and more efficient health sector have long been recognized in Europe.

Healthcare systems are becoming increasingly dependent on Information and Communication Technologies (ICTs) to deliver top-quality care to European citizens.

eHealth is an integral component of the EU's i2010[1] policy framework, which seeks to promote an open and competitive digital economy, ICT-related research, as well as applications to improve social inclusion, public services and quality of life.

At EU level, the introduction of eHealth services is facilitating access to healthcare, whatever the geographical location, thanks to innovative telemedicine and personal health systems. eHealth is also breaking down barriers, enabling health service providers (public authorities, hospitals) from different regions to work more closely together.

Hospitals, for example, in the EU seem well connected: 98% have Internet access, 78% broadband.

Some of the challenges are:

♦ The demographic changes—today, citizens aged 65+ make up close to 18 % of the total population in all EU countries, and the percentage of elderly will increase further in the following years. The most dramatic raise is expected in the 80+ age range. Aging of the population together with unhealthy lifestyles are generating an increased prevalence of chronic conditions that place additional strains on both health and social support systems. By 2050, one-third of the population will be over 60. More people will require prolonged care.

♦ Citizens' expectations for high-quality care

♦ The increased prevalence of chronic diseases, which is a substantial part of the overall healthcare costs

♦ The medical accidents and errors

♦ The staff shortages in healthcare

♦ The rising healthcare costs. Health expenditure represents more than 8.5% of GDP and grows at 4% a year (faster than the EU economic growth). It could reach 16% of GDP by 2020.

In 2004, the European Commission adopted an Action Plan that covers everything from electronic prescriptions and health cards to new information systems that reduce waiting times and errors to facilitate a more harmonious and complementary European approach to eHealth (IP/04/580).[2] It comprises three target areas:

♦ How to address common challenges and create the right framework to support eHealth;

♦ Pilot actions to jump start eHealth delivery; and

♦ Sharing best practices and measuring progress.

As a result, all Member States put in place strategies to accelerate e-Health deployment (www.ehealth-era.org). eHealth also forms an important part of the European Union's strategic framework "i2010—A European Information Society for growth and employment."[3] It focuses on the three crucial areas of a European health information space, innovation in all eHealth initiatives, and enabling greater access, involvement and inclusion of Europe's citizens and other stakeholders in healthcare provision through electronic means.

eHealth is also part of the Lead Market initiative for innovation launched by the Commission in 2008 (IP/08/12).[4] The ministerial conference on eHealth 2009 during the Czeck Presidency in February 2009 (EU2009.CZ) ended with the adoption of the Prague Declaration[5], which calls for European Member States and the European Commission to move forward on telemedicine deployment by building up confidence and trust and by removing legal barriers. The Prague Declaration which has been prepared in cooperation with the EU Member States and commented within the i2010 Subgroup on eHealth declared that it is crucial that the benefits of eHealth applications and services are further enhanced and properly distributed among all the relevant stakeholders:

♦ **eHealth for Individuals** (patients and healthcare professionals alike). For individuals, eHealth brings new possibilities in terms of increasing quality and effectiveness of services. eHealth provides new tools to take care of patients with chronic diseases. Within the European context, it can facilitate implementation of cross-border healthcare and contribute to the continuity of care.

♦ **eHealth for Society** *For society*, eHealth represents a challenge for interoperability, e-literacy, and accessibility of new technologies. It also presents great opportunities for research and development. The Lead Market Initiative earmarked eHealth sector as one of the strategic areas with high growth and innovation potential.

♦ **eHealth for Economy** eHealth offers solutions that can bring enormous savings. If properly deployed, eHealth could contribute to the transformation of the health sector and change substantially business models of healthcare facilities. These issues are gaining in importance in the current economic climate, putting increased pressure for delivery and cost efficiency in all sectors of the economy, the health sector being no exception.

E-health is currently the fastest growing industry of health sector estimated at €20 billion, i.e. 2% of health expenditure. It has the potential to more than double in size, almost reaching the volume of the market for medical devices or half the size of the pharmaceuticals market. By the end of 2010, a double digit growth rate of up to 11% is foreseen for ehealth, driven by a search for more productivity and performance. (Source: datamonitor 2007—Trends to watch: Healthcare technology).

The Commission is investing €163m in e-health research in 2009-2010. The funding is channelled through its framework seven funding call. The investment is supporting e-health services based on broadband for telemedicine.

However, speaking by video link to the e-Health 2009 conference in Prague, the Commissioner Viviane Reding said the current economic crisis facing Europe had not deterred investment in e-health research but "put the long-term benefits of e-health into sharp focus."

The Commissioner mentioned that the European economic recovery plan had already committed €1 billion of investment to make broadband universally available, and this would provide a vital spur to e-health.

Commissioner Reding emphasized also that the current economic challenges made it clearer that ever "we need to continue on e-health action plan." She concluded: "I am confident we can realise dream of European e-health action space."

As part of the work to implement the eHealth action plan,[6] the EU has commissioned a set of studies on issues, including the exchange of good practices in eHealth, how to address common challenges; patient identity in eHealth; legal and regulatory aspects of eHealth; and the impact of ICT on patient safety and risk management in healthcare. These studies are particularly focused on identifying specific areas of eHealth work that is concentrating in EU research funding under the Seventh Framework Programme.[7]

As the EU market is fragmented, there is a real challenge in standardisation and interoperability.

In this context, projects have been launched by the European Commission, such as European Patients Smart Open Services, epSOS (previously known as S.O.S., "Smart Open Services," an Open eHealth initiative for a large-scale European pilot of patient summary and electronic prescription), which is a Europewide project organized by 27 beneficiaries representing 12 EU-member states, including 6 ministries of health, 15 national competence centres and 31 companies. This makes it the first European eHealth project clustering such a large number of countries in practical cooperation.

The overarching goal of epSOS is to develop a practical eHealth framework and an Information & Communication Technology (ICT) infrastructure that will enable secure access to patient health information, particularly with respect to basic patient summaries and ePrescriptions between different European healthcare systems. There is 11 Million € EC funding for this project.

The project is co-financed by the European Commission within the Competitiveness and Innovation Programme[8] (CIP).[9] epSOS was launched on July 1, 2008, and will be in progress for 36 months.

Another example is the project CALLIOPE that has been set up by the EU-funded Thematic Network. "CALLIOPE—Creating a European coordination network for eHealth interoperability implementation."[10] The project was launched on 1 June 2008 with a duration of 30 months. It covers 23 beneficiaries with 500K€ EC funding.

E-Health is working when ehealth tools are combined with the right organisation and skills.

The following sites—www.good-ehealth.org, www.ehealth-impact.org, and www.epractice.eu—provide hundreds of successful projects that can be then disseminated in all Europe.

In Denmark, the national and regional health information networks improve quality and efficiency and save €80 Mil/Year (Medcom).

In Sweden, ePrescription improves patient safety and saves €70Mil/Year.

In UK, personal Health Systems and telemonitoring can provide care at the point of need and reduce length of hospitalisation by 20-40% for heart patients.

Direct Online Information Services, such as NHS direct online in UK, empowers patients, helping them avoid unnecessary hospitalisation and support lifestyle choices. It saves €110 Mil/Year.

Hospitals in Germany can save up to €1,5 Bill/Year through early discharge of patients made possible by mobile monitoring services (source Gesundheit Scout 24 GmbH & Bayerishes Rutes Krenz).

The €2.2m EU-funded project, which has been developed by the Estonian e-Health Foundation, aims to provide patients with a cross-country e-registration system that lists all the doctors and health services in Estonia. Estonia's national e-health strategy calls for the full implementation of by 2013.

A European Commission Analysis shows the main national priorities in Europe:

Chart 1. *National Priorities: Preliminary Analysis*

Priorities in National eHealth Strategies	# of Countries	Examples
Electronic Health Records EHR, EPR, Medical Records Patient Summary Emergency Data Set	17	DMP—Dossier Médical Personnel (FR) BEHR—Basic Structure for the EHR (DK) NHS Care Records Service/Spine (UK) Patient summary (SE, FI) SumEHR (BE) eGP file (NL)
Infrastructures & Networks Broadband communication networks and associated technology and basic services	12	MedCom—the Danish Healthcare Data Nework (DK) Sjunet (SE) National Health Network (NO) National eHealth VPN (DE, AT)
ePrescription Management and implementation of ePrescribing	16	Apotheket (SE) ePrescription (DK, NL, SI) eRezept (DE)

http://www.ehealth-era.org/

Among some other challenges that the Commission should encourage and facilitate are:

♦ The legal and regulatory barriers, such as security and privacy. A legal framework with some EU Directives is already in place, such as a Directive on personal data protection, a Directive on Information Society Services, and Electronic Commerce and Privacy-enhancing technologies. But, more should be done.

♦ Sustainable new business models and financing through private/public partnerships.

♦ User acceptance through dissemination.

♦ Extensive co-operation among stakeholders in health services and the medical professions, who often have little previous experience of international co-operation, is vital if the EU is to build a European eHealth Area and move away from fragmented delivery systems.

eHealth requires a vision and should be a way to redesign healthcare built on member states' solutions and user needs.

DR. ALAN R. SHARK is the executive director/CEO of the Public Technology Institute (PTI). He also serves as Assistant Professor at Rutgers University's School of Public Affairs and Administration. As an author, lecturer, and speaker on technology developments and applications for most of his distinguished career, Dr. Shark's experience both balances and embraces the business, government, education and technology sectors. His most recent books, *CIO Leadership for Cities & Counties—Emerging Trends & Practices* and *Beyond e-Government & e-Democracy: A Global Perspective* are available online. Dr. Shark is a Fellow of the National Academy of Public Administration (NAPA), as well as Fellow of the Radio Club of America (RCA), and Fellow of the American Society for Association Executives (ASAE). Dr. Shark holds a doctorate in Public Administration from the University of Southern California's Washington Public Policy Center.

DR. SYLVIANE TOPORKOFF is partner and founder of ITEMS International, a company specialized on strategic ICT consulting, and full Professor at the University of Paris 8, Institute of European Studies, in France. She obtained her doctorate in Economics from the University of Paris I Pantheon Sorbonne. Dr. Toporkoff is specialized on international (Europe, USA and worldwide) research and consulting in the area of the Information Society; public policy; economic and strategic international partnerships for industrialists, operators and local authorities; marketing on issues related to e-Business; e-Gov; e-health; local, regional and international development through the use of ICT; e-Democracy; and telecommunications industry regulation. Dr. Toporkoff is President and founder of the Global Forum/Shaping the Future, a think tank on ICT, which annually assembles international top-level managers of leading companies and organizations, cities and regions since 1992. The Global Forum—a not-for-profit initiative of Items International and the Sophia Antipolis Foundation—is dedicated to business and policy issues affecting the successful evolution of the Information Society. Dr. Toporkoff is "Chevalier of the Legion of Honour" and obtained the medal of "Arts, Sciences and Letters."

ENDNOTES

1. http://ec.europa.eu/information_society/eeurope/i2010/index_en.htm

2. http://europa.eu/rapid/pressReleasesAction.do?reference=IP/04/580&
   format=HTML&aged=1&language=EN&guiLanguage=en

3. http://ec.europa.eu/information_society/eeurope/i2010/docs/
   communications/com_229_i2010_310505_fv_en.pdf

4. http://europa.eu/rapid/pressReleasesAction.do?reference=IP/08/12&
   format=HTML&aged=0&language=EN&guiLanguage=en

5. http://www.ehealth2009.cz/Pages/108-Prague-Declaration.html

6. http://ec.europa.edu/information_society/doc/qualif/health/
   COM_2004_0356_F_EN_ACTE.pdf

7. http://cordis.europa.eu/fp7/home_en.html

8. http://ec.europa.eu/cip/index_en.htm

9. http://www.epsos.eu/glossary.html?txa21glossary%5Buid%5D=522&
   tx_a21glossary%5Bback%5D=3&cHash=e91ee6d5b9

10. http://www.calliope-network.eu/Portals/11/assets/documents/
    200901calliope_factsheet.pdf

Chapter 2

The Patient: Ultimate Casualty of an Ineffective Health Care System

Judith A. Carr, Ph.D., Founder & CEO, Envision Consulting, LLC

Alisoun Moore, Director of Health and Human Services for Commercial, State and Local, Northrop Grumman

Judith A. Carr, Ph.D., Founder & CEO, Envision Consulting, LLC

Alisoun Moore, Director of Health and Human Services for Commercial, State and Local, Northrop Grumman

"Physician, help yourself: thus help your patient too. Let this be his best help: that he may behold with his eyes the man who heals himself."

—FRIEDRICH NIETZSCHE

The ultimate casualty of an ineffective health care system is the patient. In an industry focused on financial viability and the bottom line, the patient experience is the by-product of inefficiency and inattention. Two key factors contribute to the abysmal state of affairs: 1) The health care industry has yet to fully embrace technology in designing and streamlining processes to support a patient-focused system; and 2) Many health care professionals lack the organizational competencies necessary to drive a patient-centric philosophy and transform the industry from an organizational rather than a medical perspective.

This chapter explores health care through the eyes of the patient and offers an innovative solution for creating a patient-centric health care system. Once the transformational vision has been defined, the challenge becomes one of strategy and implementation. We posit that the key to success lies in the creation of a hybrid set of competencies that blend medical and organizational capabilities and leverages technology on behalf of the ultimate consumer—the patient. Ultimately, e-Health transformation will require a new generation of hospital executives groomed to optimize technology and redefine health care from the perspective of the patient.

Case Study: The Human Cost of a Broken Health Care System

My father and I had a pact—he promised to live 100 years. I always envisioned my father's passing as quiet and peaceful. It would be a beautiful summer day in the sleepy little town of my birth—Wenatchee, Washington. He would start the day sharing a cup of coffee with my mother, the love of his life and wife of 66 years. He would spend the morning in his beloved garden, working his magic growing summer vegetables in the unforgiving clay that lay at the foot of the Cascade Mountains. He was supposed to fall asleep peacefully to awaken before his Maker after a long and gentle life dedicated to the woman he loved, his children, and grandchildren. Instead, my father was destined to die a painful and agonizing death far away from the valley he loved so much.

His story is not unique. Like thousands of others, he fell prey to a health care system that is inadequate, mismanaged, and focused too intently on the bottom line. His story is very poignant for me. I watched as he bravely endured the excruciating pain resulting from the prostate cancer that spread to his spine. The tragedy is that he didn't have to spend his final months in pain and suffering. A simple PSA (prostate-specific antigen) blood test costing $44 would have identified the cancer and allowed for early treatment and an optimistic prognosis. My father was the victim of a health care system designed to enhance profitability—not patient care.

With tears in his eyes, my father's physician of over 20 years admitted that per AMA protocol, he discontinued PSA testing when my father turned 75. "Most men will die of something else before the cancer gets them." My father was not advised that testing had been discontinued until his cancer had advanced to Stage 4 and his fate was sealed. Statistically, my father had defied the odds and lived long enough to die at the merciless hand of a viscous killer. The irony of my father's story is that to save a small investment in early detection, the total cost of end of life care climbed to nearly half a million dollars!

The saga of my father's end of life medical care highlights the inadequacy of the medical system and illuminates key processes that are ripe for e-Health reform. His ordeal provided my epiphany—my understanding of just how flawed the medical system is and how enhancing the "organizational" capability of health care could streamline the system and enhance the patient experience.

My father's final journey through the health care system began in the overcrowded emergency room of a suburban Maryland hospital. The waiting room, hallways, and examination rooms looked like a war zone, littered with a myriad of sick and injured people of all ages and walks of life. We quickly learned that many lacked insurance and the only portal for care was through the ER doors. Triage determined who was seen and who was destined to wait hours in the jungle of human suffering before being ushered back to the coveted examination rooms. The elderly fell at the bottom of the priority listing. My 95 year-old father waited in excruciating pain for 26 hours before he was admitted for care.

He sat for six hours, stooped over in an uncomfortable wheel chair stashed in the corner of a hallway, while I continued as his advocate to inquire where he was in the queue. I learned that positioning changed with each addition to the patient jungle and that the processes to manage the queue were grossly inadequate from both an administrative and technical perspective. Nobody owned being in charge—there was no "go to" person to find out the status of any given patient. Periodically a technician would show up to take an X-ray or draw blood for testing. Other than these brief encounters with hospital staff, waiting in the jungle was a lonely, isolating, and painful experience.

I learned that the key to getting through the system was to assume the role of "vocal" advocate. My continued inquiries eventually earned my father the luxury of being moved to a gurney in the hall, a narrow passageway cluttered with equipment and scurrying attendants. Eight hours into the ordeal, we met our first "patient advocate"—the result of my increasingly vocal inquiries as to why a 95 year-old patient was still in the hall. The patient advocates were administrators tasked with quieting the roar of the patient jungle. I learned from the patient advocate that the system was sorely lacking for the elderly and infants. This was validated as I looked back at the jungle to see several elderly patients slumped over in pain as my father had been a few hours before. I was grateful that my father could finally lie down.

Several hours later, we were moved into an examination room. We thought the ordeal had come to its conclusion. Little did we know that my father would spend the night in the examination room, ensuring that the room would be tied up for another 12 or 13 hours—the domino theory of inefficiency dictated the pace and flow for the patient jungle.

I slept by my father's side in a painfully uncomfortable chair because after twelve hours into the process, I had come to realize that my father could not navigate the system without my advocacy. The sheer numbers of patients entering through the ER had brought the system to its knees. It was painfully clear that the processes were broken and the victims were the patients. Half in jest, I asked the nurse if anyone had died waiting to be seen—it was sobering to learn that they had. I was grateful that my father was not included among them.

At long last my father was admitted to a room. It was actually pretty nice—a private room with a bathroom and a small sofa for the exhausted advocate. Again, we thought the ordeal was over. It was here that we learned that the issues were systemic to the hospital and not isolated to the ER. The caregivers were clearly stretched to the max, victims of the dysfunctional system that provided their livelihood.

Assuming the role of 24-hour advocate provided advantages and disadvantages. I could oversee the process to ensure that my father received some level of care, but I became the target of wrath for one overworked attendant. After 26 hours of waiting, I had become a strong believer in the "do no harm" philosophy. Early on, we called the nurse to unhook my father from his IV and other tubing so he could journey to the bathroom. The nurse was busy so I walked my father to the bathroom and closed the door so he could have some privacy. He was so wobbly that he fell and bumped his head. This was before I realized just how desperately ill he was. The nurse made absolutely no effort to help my father. She screamed at me—"If you stay here you have to take care of him. We are too busy." Those were not words I wanted to hear—my four advanced degrees did not include nursing!! The system was broken, and the hospital personnel were accidental victims along with the patients.

Health care technology has been the focus of significant debate and discussion. Our hospital ordeal highlighted an array of significant issues. The prescription process was legend. For example, my father required pain medication. Bone cancer is brutal, and as the disease progresses so does the level of medication. The hospital process required that the nurse enter the request into a system that generated a FAX to the pharmacy. The pharmacy then located the doctor to get approval to fill the prescription. The request then went into the queue to be filled in the order it was submitted. Once I became aware of the process, I timed a request for pain pills. It took six hours before the pill was given to my father. When I questioned the process, the nurse said that was a reasonable amount of time—after all the system was broken. They were expecting new technology, but she didn't know how soon it would be implemented. It was pretty telling that the nursing staff had become so hardened to the suffering this process caused for the patient.

On the final day of the stay, I sought out the nurse to provide some function for my father. He told me that he was four hours behind in entering data into the computer. He directed me to the cabinet and asked if I would mind taking care of my father so he could finish his administrative duties. Four "hospitalists" (on-staff physicians) appeared for random visits over the week's stay but no single person owned my father's care. The collective wisdom after thousands of dollars of testing was that my 95-year old father was terminal. With great sadness and reluctant acceptance, he was released to die in Hospice in my home.

As an organizational consultant, it was obvious to me that the system was broken both from a process and technology perspective, and the victims were the patients, their families, and the health care providers themselves. The epiphany coming out of my father's story is that the dysfunctional health care system could be improved by applying an organizational paradigm for creating effective and efficient organizations and designing technical systems to support the new process flows. In order for this to happen, health care executives must embrace a hybrid set of competencies that blend medical and organizational capabilities and leverages technology on behalf of the ultimate consumer—the patient.

I don't have the power to change my father's experience but I am committed to applying my organizational skills to fixing a system so the next father entering a hospital will have a better, more humane experience.

In Loving Memory of my father John Conrad—Judy Carr

State of the Industry

> *"Though physician to others, yet himself full of sores."*
> —LATIN PROVERB

The United States health care system is in disarray. To label it a "system" is to imply that the myriad components work in unison to achieve a common mission. Optimally, a collaborative system of health care partners would provide a strategic enterprise approach to cost-effective, patient-centric medical services. Quite the opposite is true. The system is highly fragmented—a loose configuration of insurers, payers, and providers, operating under an antiquated cottage industry model where each entity is paid for piecework by way of office visits, procedures, and tests. The greater the volume sold, the greater the revenue. The quality of what is sold as measured in the health outcome is not factored into this economic equation. As a matter of fact, it could be said that poor quality is rewarded with the need for additional office visits, procedures, and tests— all at additional cost. The current industry model is the total antithesis of a highly connected, interactive, cost effective patient-centric service delivery model.

Much has been written about deficiencies of the health care system. It is not the purpose of this chapter to opine the inadequacies of the system but to highlight key areas, if addressed, could lead to the transformation of the industry. The state of the health care industry is influenced by multiple critical success factors. For the purpose of this discussion, we will highlight two key elements driving the dysfunctional nature of the current state of affairs:

- ◆ Escalating cost of a dysfunctional health care system.
- ◆ Inadequate technical systems to support key processes.

Escalating Cost of a Dysfunctional Health Care System—The cost of health care has increased dramatically over the last forty years (see Table 1). National Health Care Expenditures (NHE) have exceeded economic growth in every decade since the 1970s, growing at an average annual rate of 9.6 percent since 1970, or 2.4 percentage points faster than nominal Gross Domestic Product (GDP). "The persistence of this trend suggests systemic differences between health care and other economic sectors where growth rates are typically more in line with overall growth" (Kaiser 2009). The key question facing those who seek to transform the health care industry is why are health care costs rising at a rate significantly higher than any other industry? If we can gain insight into the causes driving up the cost of health care, we can logically apply the organizational constructs to reverse the escalation trend.

Table 1. *Rising Cost of Health Care.*

Indicator—United States	1960s	2007
National Health Care Expenditures (NHE)	5.2% Gross Domestic Product (GDP)	16.2 % Gross Domestic Product (GDP)
Per Capita Spending on Health Care	$148	$7,421

A key factor fueling NHE, and what distinguishes health care from other economic sectors, is the degree to which costs to patients are subsidized. According to the 2009 Kaiser report, private insurance and public programs at the federal, state, and local levels now account for over 80 percent of NHE. The federal share of total spending was only 10 percent in 1964, the year prior to the creation of Medicare and Medicaid (Goldman & McGlynn 2005). Out-of-pocket spending per person as a percentage of total spending has declined since 1960, from over 50 percent to about 15 percent in 2002. As a result, Devon Herrick, Senior Fellow at the National Center for Policy Analysis, contends that "the economic incentive for patients is to consume medical services until they are worth only 14 cents on the dollar," that is, until patients have to spend their own money (Herrick 2005).

A second critical factor driving up the cost of health care is the aging population and the diseases associated with an increasingly elderly demographic. Those 65 and older account for over 12 percent of the population, up from eight percent in 1950 and four percent in 1900. The fastest growing demographic are those 85 and older (Goldman & McGlynn 2005). Those 65 and older spent on average $12,271 per person in 2000; those under age 65 spent on average $2,761 per person (Goldman & McGlynn 2005). The prevalence of disease related specifically to the aging population is a key factor in cost escalation. As the Baby Boomers come of age, health care costs will rise exponentially, further straining an already burdened system.

The piecework payment model fueled by public and private insurers creates a system whose cost growth has no breaks. The current U.S. health care delivery model may have outlived or soon will outlive our ability to pay for it and now demands a more rational model.

Inadequate Technical Systems to Support Key Processes—Historically, health care organizations have operated along functional lines, in silo fashion, with little regard to the impact on other departments up and down the care continuum (HFMA 2003). Technology decisions are, for the most part, driven by the needs of individual silo units rather than a rational system-wide IT governance process allowing for an enterprise IT architecture and standardized technologies driving cross-unit optimization, information sharing, and interoperability of systems.

As trite as it may sound, many technology decisions are random-based and influenced heavily by very effective vendor presentations of their latest technology "solutions." Many of these solutions are "out-of-the-box" and do not take into account the complex requirements or processes of individual health care organizations, let alone interoperability between organizations. They are costly, often difficult to implement, and may fail to be adopted if the out-of-the-box solution fails to fit seamlessly into the already complex workflow of busy clinics.

As a result, it is extremely difficult and often disruptive to force fit these solutions into a life/death culture that already stretches health care resources to the limit. The random selection of technologies often creates a whole array of issues that negatively impact productivity rather than streamlining an already stressed system. A 2008 Gartner survey shows that nearly two-thirds of health care chief technology officers (CIOs) site deficiencies in their enterprise governance system as a critical issue driving up the cost of health care technology (Shaffer 2008). But alas, shifting health care technology decision-making from silo to an enterprise perspective is an onerous task and not one that can easily be accomplished as a short-term solution. Compounding this issue, many health care organizations are not seamlessly hierarchal, but rather complex decentralized institutions where an enterprise approach is difficult to implement—despite its many advantages for patient care. Although it is critical for the long-term viability of the health care community to create an enterprise framework for driving mission outcomes, it is equally as important to deliver short-term options that streamline and automate processes to deliver patient-centric care and enhance the financial bottom line.

Technology is a viable means by which to achieve quick hits in terms of automating and streamlining existing processes. In addition to enterprise-wise fragmentation, the processes and technologies supporting individual units are disjointed and inefficient, resulting in underutilized assets, poor performance, and unrealized profits. The Healthcare Financial Management Association (HFMA 2003) cites the lack of an enterprise-wide care delivery system integrating data and processes of many key areas as the culprit driving a dysfunctional system (HFMA 2003).

Process integration as it relates to the operating room provides a good example of the impact fragmentation has on the patient and the bottom line. Per HFMA statistics, the average operating room (OR) runs at only 68 percent capacity. Increasing throughput by a single additional procedure per day per OR suite can generate anywhere from $4 million to $7 million in additional annual revenue for the average-sized organization (HFMA 2003). Patients are backed up in queues waiting for their turn in the OR or worse yet, have to be rescheduled because the resources did not converge in time for their procedures.

Understanding the OR from a holistic care-delivery perspective based on the interdependence of each sequenced component in the process is essential to streamlining OR events. The challenge for hospitals is that many steps in the process (e.g., scheduling, supply selection and usage, and sequencing OR turnover) are performed manually and, therefore, lack any level of standardization. The lack of standardization makes it incredibly difficult to effect meaningful process management. The key to turning around this deplorable situation is to standardize the processes and effect workflow automation. Two immediate benefits will include improved efficiencies and decision-making and freeing of skilled nurses from manual functions to spend more time enhancing patient care (HFMA 2003).

Process Integration & Workflow Automation Advantages (HFMA)

- ◆ Improved profits
- ◆ Performance management improvements
- ◆ Maximized resource utilization
- ◆ Streamlined work flow
- ◆ Supply cost reductions
- ◆ Enhanced care delivery

In terms of optimizing health care technology, a tandem approach to technology implementation should include a strategic long-term vision and framework driving enterprise level change and a tactical shorter-term approach of achieving workflow efficiencies through the automation of manual processes.

Vision for a Patient-Centric Health Care System

"Restore a man to his health, his purse lies open to thee."
—Robert Burton

In the late nineties, both business and government transformed their operational models using information technology (IT) to shift to net-centric models, most notably the Internet. The transformation was a quiet revolution giving birth to innovative citizen/customer-centric business models that allowed for direct online service delivery. This quiet revolution drove incredible cost savings to both consumer and business alike. The paradigm shift was dramatic—changing the focus from tactical backend IT processes to using IT to craft entirely new service delivery models. The new IT model required a fully integrated business model.

Health care has yet to fully embrace the IT paradigm. While there have been dramatic improvements in some areas of health IT such as state-of-the-art MRI machines, patient centric workflow systems have been slow to arrive. In fact, adoption of the basic components of patient centric systems such as electronic medical records, e-prescribing, computerized physician order entry systems (CPOE) and web-based access to physicians, appointment scheduling tests, and records has been extremely slow. Many IT innovations have focused solely on improving back end institution-centric processes, not patient-centric or, dare we say, customer-centric processes. The health care industry continues to operate in silo fashion, failing to optimize systems that drive cross-organizational transparency. As we look to the future of health care, it is obvious that technology will play a central role in driving new business practices and enhanced patient care.

Crafting a vision that is inclusive for all health care organizations is a daunting task. Each organization has its own unique mission and challenges and falls at a different place along the continuum between well run and dysfunctional. For the purpose of this discussion, we look to the research sponsored by The Joint Commission Public Policy Initiative to find common ground and a universal vision for the health care industry (2008).

> *In a nutshell, the vision for tomorrow's health care industry is to design and implement a cost-effective system of providing patient-centric services, utilizing new business and service delivery models and optimizing health care IT.*

The United States health care industry finds itself at a crossroad—to continue down a path where per capita health care spending is more than 50 percent higher than any other country (Anderson & Hussey 2005) and patient satisfaction is at an all time low, or transforming the industry through the adoption of creative business models and innovative technologies.

Volumes have been written about the state of the US health care industry and the requirements for an industry turn around. It is not the purpose of this discussion to further dialog the elements of an industry vision but to focus more on the executive competencies that will be required to lead the monumental change initiative. Suffice it to say, highlighting the key areas requiring guiding principles for decision-making is a critical first step in creating the future state of the health care industry (see Health Care Vision below). The framework has been established to envision the future state and debate the options for achieving the required outcomes.

Health Care Vision Guiding Principles (The Joint Commission)

- ◆ Support economic viability
- ◆ Guide technology adoption
- ◆ Guide achievement of patient-centered care
- ◆ Address staffing challenges
- ◆ Guide design

Strategy for Transformation

"A physician who treats himself has a fool for a patient."
—WILLIAM OSLER

Transformation of the health care industry is no small task. It will require next generation paradigms to redefine key issues including service delivery models and patient care. A critical component of crafting and implementing a viable transformation strategy is to redefine the competencies required to catapult health care into the future. Historically, heath care issues have been addressed by health care executives—promulgating the paradigm that only those inside the industry can drive change. Traditional heath care competencies alone have proven to be ineffective in stemming the tide of escalating costs and poor patient care.

Next Generation Health Care Paradigm

Transformation requires the convergence of health care and organizational competencies. The health care industry must decide whether to grow organizational competencies internally or partner with organizational experts to drive transformational change.

The predominance of health care executives come from the physician or nursing communities and have had little or no formal training or experience driving large-scale change. Transformation of the magnitude required demands a paradigm shift – one that merges health care and organizational competencies. The missing link in the existing system is a well-developed organizational perspective.

The time has come to introduce a new paradigm that can effectively address an innovative strategy for revamping the health care system. Figure 1 identifies: 1) the vision or requirements of the future state, 2) the competencies required to drive transformation, and 3) the outcomes to be achieved by implementing the new health care paradigm. The Model for Health Care Transformation provides the framework for discussing issues and options.

The vision for the health care industry can be described as *health care by design*. The concept is simple in its fundamental premise that significant change should be driven by informed decisions based on fundamental principles. The Joint Commission (2008) has identified five critical components of the health care vision (see Figure 1) and has crafted a set of principles for each. It falls to health care executives to orchestrate the vision and actualize the required outcomes.

Figure 1. *Health Care Transformation.*

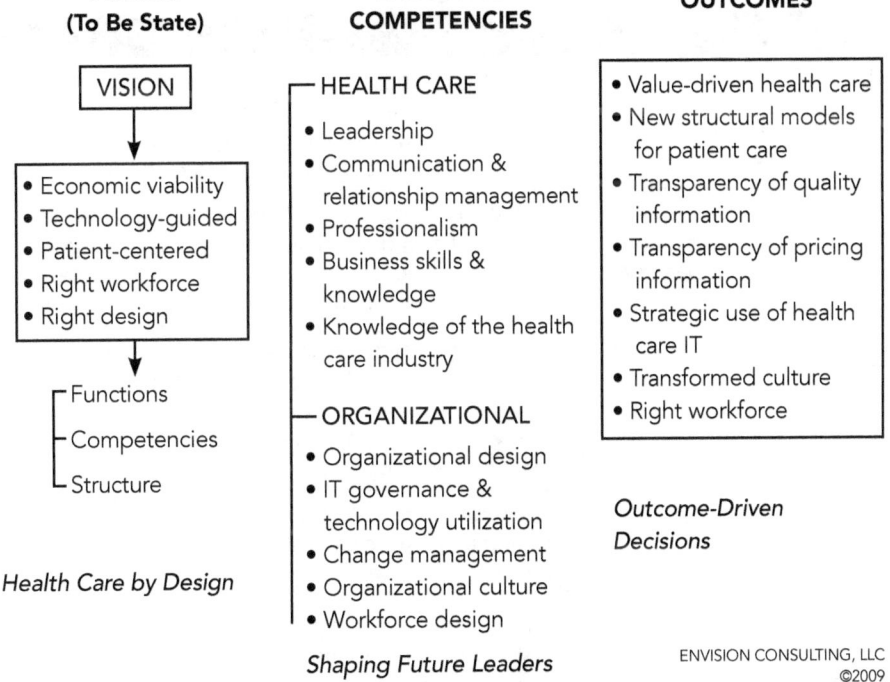

FUTURE (To Be State)

VISION

- Economic viability
- Technology-guided
- Patient-centered
- Right workforce
- Right design

- Functions
- Competencies
- Structure

Health Care by Design

EXECUTIVE COMPETENCIES

HEALTH CARE

- Leadership
- Communication & relationship management
- Professionalism
- Business skills & knowledge
- Knowledge of the health care industry

ORGANIZATIONAL

- Organizational design
- IT governance & technology utilization
- Change management
- Organizational culture
- Workforce design

Shaping Future Leaders

OUTCOMES

- Value-driven health care
- New structural models for patient care
- Transparency of quality information
- Transparency of pricing information
- Strategic use of health care IT
- Transformed culture
- Right workforce

Outcome-Driven Decisions

ENVISION CONSULTING, LLC
©2009

We believe that the enabling executive competencies fall into two categories—traditional health care competencies and organizational competencies. The traditional competencies provide general capabilities and form the foundation for current operations and tactical change, whereas the organizational competencies provide the framework for driving strategic change. Both are critical to the future of health care and both contribute to achieving the required outcomes. With the convergence of traditional health care competencies and organizational competencies comes the next generation health care paradigm—*health care by design.*

Health Care Competencies—Health care competencies have been defined by many constituency groups. For the purpose of this discussion, we will use the five families of competencies defined by The American College of Health Care Executives (ACHE 2008). See Table 2 for definitions. The first four competencies tend to be more generic by definition and although they create a framework for change, they do not generate the capability required to redefine an industry. The business skills and knowledge family of competencies addresses key areas such as systems thinking, organizational dynamics and governance, information management, and quality improvement, and as such provides the bridge to a more organization-centered approach to health care management. The key

Table 2. *Health Care Competencies (ACHE 2008).*

Competency	Definition
Leadership	The ability to inspire individual and organizational excellence, create a shared vision and successfully manage change to attain the organization's strategic ends and successful performance.
Communication & Relationship Management	The ability to communicate clearly and concisely with internal and external customers, establish and maintain relationships, and facilitate constructive interactions with individuals and groups.
Professionalism	The ability to align personal and organizational conduct with ethical and professional standards that include a responsibility to the patient and community, a service orientation, and a commitment to lifelong learning and improvement.
Knowledge of the Healthcare Environment	The understanding of the healthcare system and the environment in which healthcare managers and providers function.
Business Skills & Knowledge	The ability to apply business principles, including systems thinking, to the health care environment.

point to be made is the organizationally oriented competencies are less developed for health care executives who emerge from the medical disciplines. We contend that it is critical to grow a next generation of health care executives steeped in the theory and experience of the organizational competencies.

Organizational Competencies—Innovation by definition provides a new approach to problem solving. Viewing health care reform through an organizational lens may well be the innovative approach required to move a faltering industry closer to the cost-effective, patient-centric model required in today's environment. The purpose of the following dialog is to pique interest in a set of organizational competencies and to provide examples of how two very critical organizational competencies can play an integral role in redefining health care. We will save the exhaustive study and subsequent debate for another venue.

Organization Design—Health care organizations are exploring alternative service delivery models in an attempt to reduce costs and enhance the quality of patient care. It is critical to design innovative organizational models to deliver on the new requirements. One such model is the specialty hospital or "focused factory." The specialty hospital serves a subset of patients and performs specific procedures such as cardiac care and orthopedic surgery. Unencumbered by the need to provide general services, a specialty hospital can produce higher margins, focused expertise, and higher volume (The Joint Commission 2008). A collection of specialty hospitals rather than full service general hospitals could provide a viable option to counter the ineffective models of the past. The key point is that one model does not fit the requirements of all health care organizations.

A second phenomenon occurring in today's health care environment is the concept of "medical tourism." Patients from developed countries travel abroad to acquire high quality care at dramatically lower costs (The Joint Commission 2008). The loss of revenue to U.S. hospitals was $16 billion in 2008 and is expected to rise to $68 billion in by 2010 (Deloitte 2008). In essence, this is a hybrid version of outsourcing—one driven by the patient or customer community rather than by the organization. It begs the question of approaching outsourcing from an organizational perspective. In the pure essence of the concept, the health care community could potentially lower costs, deliver more "focused" care, and flatten organizations by selecting which services to keep and which to outsource. According to the Joint Commission report (2008), hospitals are scrambling to define partnerships enabling them to have better control over the process. Outsourcing by design requires a higher-level competency and perhaps the guidance of a skilled practitioner.

Organization design is a high level competency gleaned through years of education and experience. Organizational experts understand the nuances of design and how best to craft an organization to meet mission outcomes. They are also skilled at leading executives through the decision process to arrive at *health care by design.*

IT Governance & Technology Utilization—Health care IT (HIT) has been the focus of much political debate. The issues are legion. Manual patient records are extremely costly and inefficient, not to mention inconvenient for the patient who has to disclose his/her data multiple times in the course of a single illness. Systems created in silos do not effectively share information across organizations and silo "solutions" foster great expense in terms of cost, inefficiency, and patient inconvenience. The lack of an effective "enterprise" approach to IT has engendered soaring costs and inefficiencies. The ills of the industry cry out for an effective IT governance system to ensure that enterprise-wide IT decisions are consistent with pre-agreed upon principles and standards, and that IT is ultimately used to drive more effective business models and patient care.

Technologies, both current and future, will be used to support new service delivery models. For example, the Veteran's Administration's (VA) national Care Coordination Home Telehealth (CCHT) program has used technology to shift chronic care management from institutions to the home. This highly effective and cost effective service delivery model leverages an electronics record system that stores updated data right from the patient's home. The point to be made is this is one technology application; many more innovative technology solutions are on the horizon. It is critical that those implemented fall under the umbrella of an effective IT governance process so that the health care industry can enhance interoperability and cost-effective IT investment.

Although this competency has a strong technology focus, it requires a high-level, mission-savvy organizational person to guide the creation of a framework to support future IT capability. It is equally as important to automate the health care processes to ensure cost-effective, patient-centric service delivery. An organizational person is well equipped to understand process flow and the implications of technology-facilitated systems.

Conclusion

> *"The art of medicine consists in amusing the patient*
> *while nature cures the disease."*
> —VOLTAIRE

The case study paints a graphic picture of the experience of one elderly patient who is representative of a community suffering at the hand of an ineffective health care system. We are in the midst of a perfect storm—the convergence of critical systemic deficiencies that cry out for transformation. The health care community has come together to identify critical characteristics of the future they wish to create (e.g., economic viability, technology-guided, patient-centered, right workforce and right design). *The vision is health care by design.*

Health care by design challenges existing paradigms, implying that the vision can be orchestrated with purpose rather than happenstance. Achieving the vision is difficult and will require health care executives to leverage technology and augment health care competencies with competencies of an organizational nature. Transformation of the magnitude proposed requires a new breed of health care executive—one that is comfortable managing at the vortex of change.

The future for health care will include new cost-effective service delivery models, optimization of enterprise technologies to streamline processes and enhance the patient experience, and new approaches for reinventing a dysfunctional industry. As the industry moves closer to achieving *health care by design,* the patient will emerge as the victor in the transformation.

"Physician, help yourself: thus help your patient too."

DR. JUDY CARR, PH.D. is the founder and CEO of Envision Consulting, LLC, an executive coaching and organizational consulting firm dedicated to helping government executives achieve personal and organizational excellence. She is a recognized expert in human and organizational issues that fall at the intersection of business and technology. Judy's forte is turning theory and best practices into organizational models that are practical and measurable. Judy is the coach of choice for organizations engaged in large-scale transformation. Her recent accomplishments include designing and orchestrating a workforce transformation initiative for the U.S. Air Force and designing a cultural transformation/organizational competency initiative for Goddard Space Flight Center. As a Gartner VP, Judy served as an executive advisor to over 100 CIOs and other C-level executives. Her book, *Consumer Evolution: Nine Effective Strategies to Drive Business Growth,* has been widely used by organizations to develop client-focused service delivery models driving customer satisfaction. Judy holds a Ph.D. in Human and Organizational Systems, publishing a dissertation entitled "Human Factors: A New Perspective for Software Systems Development." She also holds a B.A. in Business Administration and Economics, an M.S. in Organization Development, and an M.A. in Human Development.

ALISOUN MOORE is the Director of Health and Human Services for Commercial, State and Local, Northrop Grumman. As director, she leads development of health and human services applications for several state and local clients. She is the former Chief Information Officer for Montgomery County, Maryland, which has about 1 million residents and is located just north of Washington, D.C. Under her leadership, the county has won numerous awards, including the Best of Web for the best national portal for a large jurisdiction. Montgomery County has also consistently placed in the top 10 of Digital Governments as ranked by the Center for Digital Government. Prior to her work at the county, Ms. Moore served as the State of Maryland's Chief Information Officer and worked on passing critical eGovernment legislation requiring state agencies to provide services online to citizens. Ms. Moore has written numerous articles, worked with the World Bank and the University of Maryland on eGovernment initiatives for developing nations, and has spoken in several countries regarding this topic. Her current interest is in applying technology to improve health care delivery and reduce costs. Ms. Moore holds a Bachelor's degree from the University at Albany in Political Science and Biology, a Masters in Public Administration with a concentration in Information Technology from the University of Baltimore and is now working on a Masters of Business Administration at Johns Hopkins University with a concentration on health care management.

REFERENCES

Anderson, Gerard, Hussey, Peter F., et al, "Health care spending in the U.S. and the rest of the industrialized world," *Health Affairs*, 24, no. 4 (2005): 903-914

Anderson, Gerard (2007). AHA Survey 2007. Retrieved from AHA website: www.aha.org/aha/content/2007/PowerPoint/StateofHospitalsChartPack2007.ppt

Branz, Kay A., Publisher (2009). ACHE Healthcare Executive Competencies Assessment Tool 2009. Healthcare Executive Magazine. Retrieved July 15, 2009 from HCHE website: www.ache.org/pdf/nonsecure/careers/competencies_booklet.pdf

Darkins, A., Ryan, P., Kobb, R., et al, "Care Coordination/Home Telehealth: The systematic implementation of health informatics, home telehealth and disease management to support the care of veteran patients with chronic conditions," *Telemedicine and e-Health*, in press

Deloitt (2008). Medical Tourism Study. Retrieved July 17, 2009 from the Deloitt website: http://www.deloitte.com/dtt/cda/doc/content/us_chs_MedicalTourismStudy(1).pdf

F., Frogner, Bianca K., et al, "Health care spending and use of information technology in OECD countries," *Health Affairs*

Herrick, Devon M. (2005, May). Consumer driven health care: the changing role of the patient. Retrieved April 14, 2009, from National Center for Policy Analysis Web site: http://www.ncpa.org/pub/st/st276

HFMA, (2003, March). Achieving Operating Room Efficiency through Process Integration.

HFMA Annual Report 2002-2003. Retrieved July 31, 2009, from McKesson Web site: http://www.mckesson.com/static_files/McKesson.com/MPT/Documents/HFMAProcessIntegration.pdf

Kaiser Family Foundation, (2009, March). Health care costs: a primer. Retrieved April 14, 2009, from Kaiser Family Foundation Web site: http://www.kff.org/insurance/upload/7670_02.pdf

Kaiser Family Foundation, (2009, February). Kaiser health tracking poll. Retrieved March 20, 2009, from Kaiser Family Foundation Web site: http://www.kff.org/kaiserpolls/upload/7866.pdf

Shaffer, Vi, (2008, September). A Benchmark of Healthcare IT Governance and Approaches for Improvement, 2008, from Gartner Web site: http://my.gartner.com/resources/161300/161392/a_benchmark_of_healthcare_it_161392.pdf?h=62F8AA029AF573B905A9DCA64A4A5E4812CC9648

Chapter 3

Learning from the Past–Preparing for the Future: On Medical Information Systems Evaluation

Ypapanti Thermou, Department of Computer Science and Biomedical Informatics, University of Central Greece

Yannis Charalabidis and Ilias Maglogiannis, Department of Information and Communication Systems Engineering, University of Aegean

Introduction

The concept of a MIS is, directly, connected with the meaning of the improvement of health services' quality that hospitals and generally caregivers provide. It is accepted that the main components of such a system concern not only organizational but also social issues. Therefore, the evaluation should approach technical and technological issues as well as organizational ones. There are three main factors under consideration: the contribution of technology, human factors and organization.

The purpose of this study is to prove that we are able to create an evaluation framework which is consisted of comprehensive measures and dimensions of a Medical Information System and promote a matching way of the referred factors. The evaluation aims at two main pillars. Firstly, it examines if a MIS meets the clinical needs, improving clinical performance and the impact of results on a patient and, secondly, it investigates the extent of acceptance by users. Nevertheless, there is a multitude of problems and challenges that should be faced by the "evaluators" [1]. For example, some may be the following: imprecise or alternating targets during the study, great effort in preparation and performance evaluation, complex or sometimes contradictory results, affected results by the user's motivations and their expectations, and, finally, the uncertainty whether the results can be generalized to other environments.

In a limited extend of this work, the quantity and quality of publications related to Medical Information Systems are mentioned. It concerns, mainly, the methods used during the evaluation and what should be the necessary components of a published evaluation so as to be considered complete and sufficient.

Theoretical Background

There is a proposed framework, called HOT-fit (Human, Organization, Technology) framework, [2, 3] that was developed after critical thought based on literature related to MIS. It aims to combine and understand the way in which human and organizational factors impact on technology and vice versa. There are two basic evaluation models which complement one another in order to establish the proposed framework. These two models are the IS Success Model and the IT-Organization Fit Model. They both have some significant factors which play a key role for the success of a system and some criteria that may lead to failure, such as low level of skills, lack of acceptance, difficult transition from the usual workflow patterns to new ones.

However, before we look at these two models, which are more comprehensive and specialized, it should be noted that several approaches [3] for evaluation have, already, developed. Various models based on plurality of structures comprise technical, social, financial and human issues. Some frameworks are presented in Table 1, where each model emphasizes at different clusters of attributes.

Table 1. *Early approaches to MIS evaluation; selected frameworks.*

Framework	Evaluation factors		
	Technology	Human	Organization
4Cs (Kaplan, 1997)	MIS and its developing impact	Communication	Control, care, context
CHEATS (Shaw, 2002)	Technical	Human, Educational, Social	Clinical, Organization, Management
TEAM (Grant, et al., 2002)	IS based on management level	Role	Structure
ITAM (Dixon, 1999)	IT adaptation	User	

IS Success Model

Having as objective the construction and representation of interactions among the research results, a comprehensive classification was proposed. It is a model which includes six categories or dimensions that are linked together and give a more dynamic presentation of how the model works.

These 6 dimensions are shown in the following figure and are as follows [2]:

1. System Quality, measures relating to procedural information of the system itself
2. Information Quality, measures for the output data
3. Service Quality, measures for the technical support and service
4. System Use, it considers whether the output information is "consumed"
5. User Satisfaction
6. Network benefits

Figure 1. *Information System Success Model.*

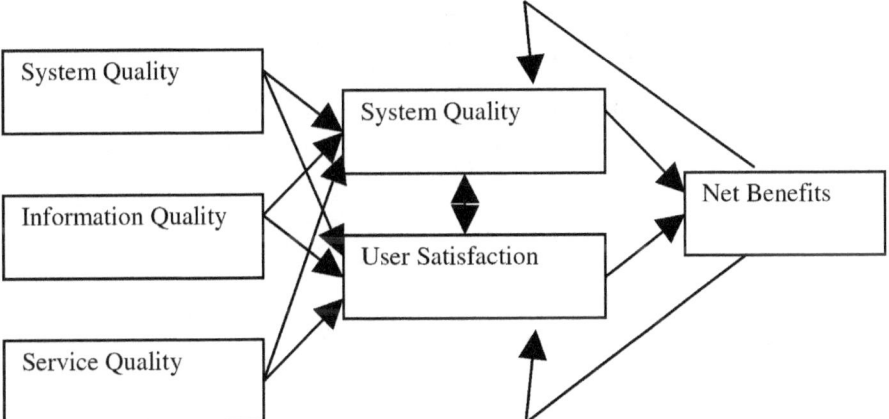

This framework is cyclical, thus, it is possible that positive or negative influence can affect each level of the model. A typical example shows the interaction between the dimension "user satisfaction" with the "use" of it. If the user handles the system in a correct way, the benefits accruing for the system promote its use and expansion. Otherwise, if there is misuse, the advantages of the system do not become apparent and thus the system is rejected.

IT-Organization Fit Model

The IT Organizational Fit Model has some similarities with the previous model but also makes a distinction between external and internal components of the system that should be taken into account. The internals concern organizational ingredients, such as strategy, organizational structure, management processes, roles and skills. External factors, on the other hand, concern the environmental trends and changes, such as market, industry and technology. This model is, also, understandable and includes three factors: technology (IT), human (roles and skills) and organization (structure, management processes) with particular emphasis on the importance of human factors. The structure of IT Organizational Fit Model is shown in Figure 2.

Figure 2. *IT–Organizational Fit Model.*

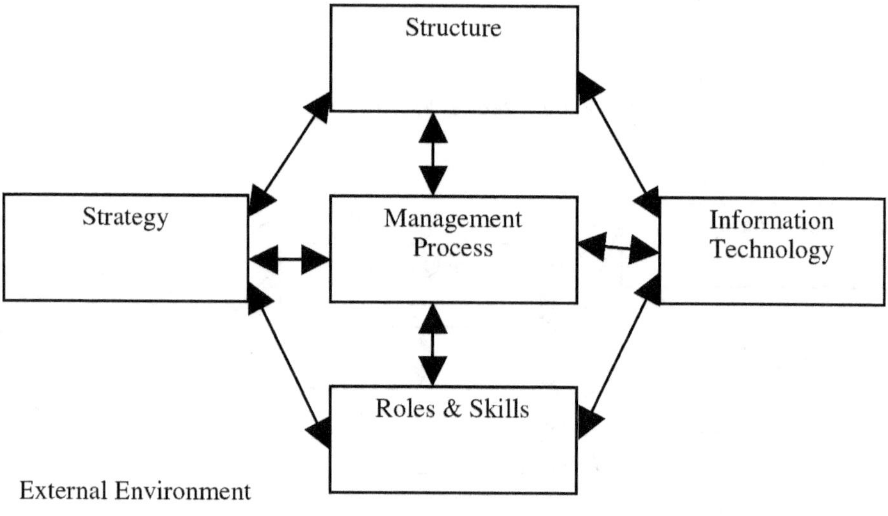

HOT-fit Framework

Taking under consideration the above two models, the researchers decided to propose a new analytical framework which would combine the features of the previous ones. Figure 3 shows the number of effects about these three factors and if this effect is one way or bidirectional. For example, we observe that the quality of services affects all measures of the human factor while they, in turn, can not wield any influence on improving the poor quality of services. Instead, the quality of exported information can affect user satisfaction and through this positive or negative influence, the user will use sound or not the system. Moreover, if the user is satisfied with the system's functions, knowing the benefits offered, it can make appropriate use leading to (better) quality information. Apart from this influence, the adaptation of these three factors (symbolized in Figure 3 marked with bold lines) is considered complex, abstract and subjective, in accordance with the strategic planning and needs. In efforts to simplify the whole evaluation system, a number of measures have used to identify specific features by clustering the dimensions human, technology, organization and benefits. Examples of these measures are shown in Table 2 and Table 3.

Figure 3. *Human-Organization-Technology Fit (HOT-fit) framework.*

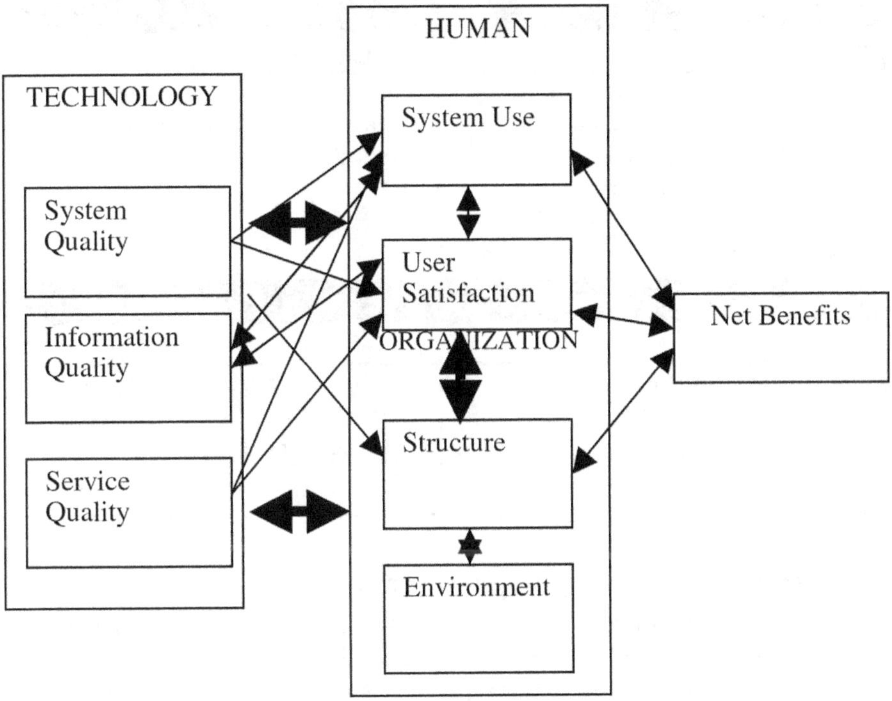

Table 2. *Examples of the proposed framework's net benefits.*

Net benefits	Clinical practice (efficiency, productivity, labor-intensive), efficiency, effectiveness (goal attainment, service), quality decision making (analysis, accuracy, participation), error reduction, clinical results (patient's care, mortality, morbidity), cost

Table 3. *Examples of the evaluation measures of the proposed framework.*

Technology		
System quality	Information quality	Service quality
easy to use, easy to learn, availability flexibility, reliability, technical support, security, response time, availability security	relevance, importance, accuracy, completeness, data input methods, quality, timeliness, availability	Quick response, precision, follow up service
Human		
System use	User Satisfaction	
Quantity/duration (number of queries, number of used functions, number of reports, frequency of report demands, number of produced reports), used by whom? Incentives for use and expansion, knowledge/skills, acceptance	Satisfaction with special functions, relevant to usefulness, satisfaction with decision making	
Organization		
Structure	Environment	
type, size, design, strategy, management, autonomy, communication, teamwork, leadership, communication	Financial source, government policy, competition, external communication, population served	

Assessment with 4 key requirements

In this section, an alternative framework is presented. It is proposed by the NCVHS (National Committee on Vital and Health Statistics) and DHHS (Department of Health and Human Services) of U.S.A [5] and also needs to have 4 requirements:

1. **Completeness of information**—All the medical information for everyone in a community belongs to a system and is accessible to all points of care.

2. **Utilization**—Relevant parts of the community that use the system -> providers and patients

3. **Type of use**—The information is used for a range of health care needs -> patient care, public health, clinical research, quality improvement.

4. **Financial support**—The implementation of IT infrastructure is financed by current income.

This framework "considers" as important to, clearly, define the targets and measures that need to be used for evaluation. Thus, guided by the 4 requirements, equivalent subcategories were created in order to collect additional information on the procedure. In each subcategory, a 5 point scale was used, where 1 represents 0-20% participation and 5 represents participation between 80-100%. For example, the first requirement divided into 8 categories, where each one is scored with a number ranging from 1 to 5, including: inpatients, outpatients, long term care, laboratory results, insurance, etc. Each category is an aggregate amount that is an average using weight coefficients. This number indicates the percentage coverage of every requirement. A similar procedure is followed in each category. The produced results are displayed at the following table (Table 4).

Table 4. *Results of the 4 requirements framework's implementation.*

	Spokane, WA	Whatcom, WA	Indianapolis, IN	South Bend, IN
Completeness of information	19/40 (48%)	21/40 (53%)	20/40 (50%)	16/40 (40%)
Degree of use	5/10 (50%)	6/10 (60%)	4/10 (40%)	4/10 (40%)
Type of use	5/5 (100%)	5/5 (100%)	5/5 (100%)	3/5 (60%)
Financial support	5/5 (100%)	5/5 (100%)	3/5 (60%)	5/5 (100%)
Total score	34/60	37/60	32/60	28/60
% total score	57%	62%	53%	47%
Weighted score (25%/sector)	74%	78%	63%	60%
Average score %	69% (8.8%)			

Evaluation Process

The methodology focuses on quantitative analysis of results [2]. Here are six basic phases of analysis. The original evaluation framework is constructed by the findings of the first phase in which the definition of existing problems and identification of users take place. Then, the research protocol is shaped based on the initial framework. In the fourth stage, data collection, analysis and reorganization are executed in order to provide documented results in the next phase. Finally, the framework is redefined taking into account the elements from the original framework and the exported results (Figure 4, see next page).

Data collection [4] is accomplished using some tools such as:

- ◆ Questionnaires
- ◆ Interviews
- ◆ Observations
- ◆ Document analysis
- ◆ Work sampling, time measurements

Case Studies

Fundus Imaging System (FIS)

The first case study concerns the Fundus Imaging System (FIS) which came with two main aims: (a) to evaluate the involved factors in implementing a specialized information system and (b) to ground the proposed framework that is discussed at unit 2.3. Furthermore, it is obvious that some factors that affect at the system should have been observed. And what could be the relationship among them in order to lead the adoption of a system in hospitals to success or failure?

This application was implemented in a primary care organization (PCO) and two cooperating special hospitals, all of them members of the National Health Service in England. This study assesses the development of a digital imaging system (FIS) for diabetic retinopathy, which can lead to blindness. The system uses a miniature camera and digital imaging software, which records images from the patients' eyes. Those patients who suffered from diabetes had to undergo a test that doctor examines patient's eye with an ophthalmoscope, to check and

Figure 4. *Research design.*

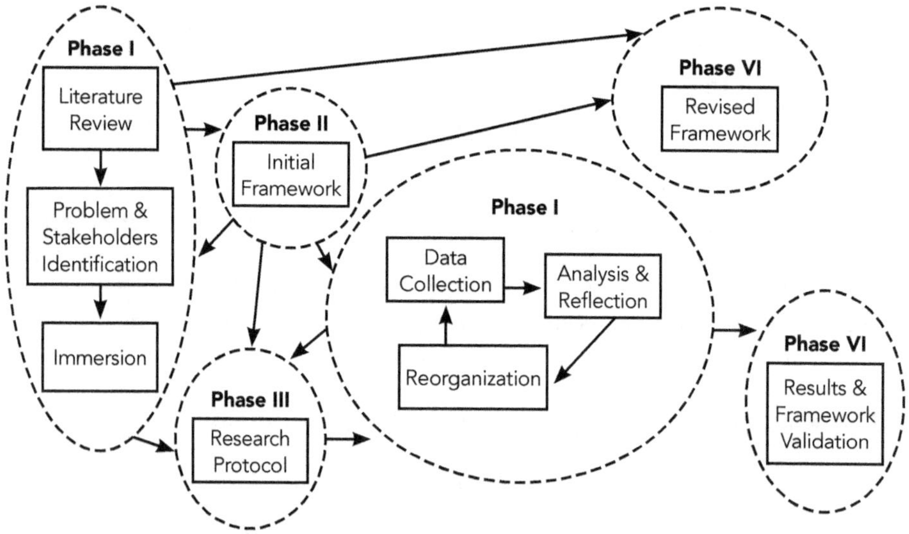

foresee the evolution of the disease by providing knowledge to patients. Essentially, during and after the examination, each patient discussed with his doctor about the results, clinical implications and how to enhance the control of diabetes, saving time since it was not necessary to fix new appointments for the analysis of results, as usual.

The used methodology consists of six phases mentioned above. For the evaluation of the FIS, the HOT-fit framework was used as driver axle and includes comments on daily clinics procedures, appointments, discussions and social events that happen in different parts of the hospital and attitudes of nurses, besides the official data collection.

As a result, all the procedures of this pilot study led to the discovery of some findings for each factor that are represented at figure 3, describing the HOT-fit framework. In terms of technological infrastructure, the study was equipped with advanced computing and telecommunications apparatus. However, some non-efficient features were observed, such as storage capacity, i.e. the files should be transferred from a small memory card (connected to the camera) to a hard disk.

Another drawback was the slow response time. For example, a doctor noted that it takes a long time to print the list of exercises for each patient (2 min), according to her view. On the other hand, there was accurate and complete data avoiding misdiagnosis results. The human factor played a decisive role here as some users had difficulties in using the system because either through ignorance of handling such systems or refusal to adopt the new application devaluing its worth and functionality.

An additional point was the difficulty of communication between the users of the system with the technical staff as the first often did not understand the terminology used by the second ones. As part of the organization, the use of new technologies giving the benefits of a new application was considered of major importance.

Finally, the results regarding the benefits of implementing the system were oriented at the quality of service, increasing the efficiency and effectiveness of clinical practice, training the patients and increasing their satisfaction.

Four assessment requirements

This evaluation framework consisted of the four requirements that was described in Subsection 2.4 was applied to four organizations that provide health care services and recorded the following results (Table 4) with use of questionnaires to the respective rates [5].

As shown in the above table, the score is between 60% to South Bend, IN, and (the highest) 78% in Whatcom, WA, with an average score of 69%. The Whatcom, WA, a 300,000 population community, has the highest rate as a result of the combination of use and cooperation from both staff and patients. It is interesting to note here that only one of the four groups which were evaluated has score greater than 75%, while there has been no assessment of the system's architecture that was installed.

Notwithstanding, in this study there is a multitude of limitations. For instance, measures related to the use of system (from doctors and patients) are rough and their replicability has to be checked, the weighting coefficients were equal to four arbitrary parameters, the degree of codification of the imported information in the form of "free" text was not evaluated and, last but by no means least, the present framework apply measures that were different from similar studies.

Evaluation of Electronic Medical Records (EMR)

The evaluation of medical information systems reflects the relationships among users, technology and the medical environment as already mentioned. This evaluation estimates not only how acceptable is from the users, something which has been emphasized in the study of the FIS, but also if it operates. The former it focuses on what we evaluate, the latter what are the potential benefits, following the model S-P-O (structure, process, output), with factors similar to those of the IS Success Model.

S-P-O: (Structure)=>(Process)=>(Outcome)

Two hospitals of South Taiwan took place to this study [6]. Hospital A that is a medical centre with more than 1,200 beds and a peripheral (educational) hospital B with about 400 general beds installed different servers and data bases but the same record system and functional strategies. This study was focused on the health professionals who need to daily handle the system. Data collected with questionnaires (61 structured questions and "free" text) in a scale from 1 to 5 ("I agree a lot," "I agree a least") and ensuant to this, the collected data was statistically analyzed with reciprocation analysis (ANOVA).

From the results presented in Table 5 we can see that there are differences in seven dimensions in the two hospitals, observing that the staff of the second was more satisfied.

Then, a revision of the model and analysis of factors took place for the initial and revised model. The results showed that the revised model was better than the original. Applying the S-P-O model they made some documentations like that technology (structure) affects the human factor (process), and man in turn

Table 5. *The results of ANOVA analysis.*

**p<a=0.01

	ANOVA	Mean—Hospital_	Mean – Hospital_
System quality	0.00**	3.14	3.50
Medical information quality	0.00**	3.35	3.61
Service quality	0.00**	2.76	3.38
Secure quality	0.00**	3.36	3.60
User's use	0.00**	3.23	3.47
User satisfaction	0.00**	3.34	3.52
Benefits	0.00**	3.30	3.52

affects the result (outcome). Finally, two cases were verified (they were statistically significant) and these are:

♦ There is no significant difference between the two hospitals, although they belong to the same organization.

♦ The existing electronic medical records need to be improved.

There are interactions between the use of the system (by the user) and the quality of medical information, user satisfaction with the quality of safety and user satisfaction with system's use, but they are not statistically significant.

Evaluation Studies

In recent decades, the application of information systems in health and the need to improve and extend their capabilities, led to a number of studies designed to evaluate or create a capable framework that could adequately describe the advantages and disadvantages of a system. Many of these studies did not follow a model but they were based on the research power of the author. According to [4], there are ten modules (Table 6, see next page) that should be described in any reference such as the introduction (problems, motivation, questions to answer), methods (collecting and analyzing data, comparisons between groups), and selection results.

This study examined 120 articles, using data from clinical units, clinics or hospital, although there is a preference in multi-hospitals, currently, as shown at the above chart. In most studies the data collection includes documents analysis (65.8%) and questionnaires (31.7%) and, generally, a 40% rate prefers to combine at least two methods of information retrieval. In short, there was improvement in the quality of evaluation studies covering more sections and providing the ability to control the reliability of methods from 1982 until 2005.

Table 6. *Ten items that should be included in reports of evaluation studies on IT interventions in health care.*

	Paper heading	Description
1	Introduction	Motivation, problems and study questions are clearly described: Does the study have a scientific basis with relevant literature references and a clear study objective?
2	Introduction/ Methods	The evaluated information technology (the intervention), is described in sufficient detail: Is the information technology under study sufficiently described including hardware, software, position of the information system in the total information infrastructure, functionality that is available and functionality that is really used, number and types of regular users, usage patterns, age/maturity of the technology, integration into workflow? Is timing and procedure of the intervention (e.g. a new IT system, a new IT function) described in sufficient details?
3	Methods	Type, number, and sampling of involved study population are clearly described: What is the unit of analysis (e.g. patients, doctors, departments)? Is the number and type of participants clearly indicated (e.g. junior physicians, only outpatient units)? How are the subjects chosen and recruited? Are inclusion and exclusion criteria clear?
4	Methods	Setting and population seem justified to answer study question: Is the unit of analysis appropriately chosen to answer the study question? Is the setting in which this study took place sufficient representative and appropriate to answer the study question?
5	Methods	Methods for collecting data are sufficiently clear: Is it clearly described how data is collected (e.g. interview, focus groups, document analysis, extraction from patient record, time measurement, etc.) and whether it was collected retrospectively or prospectively? Were validated measures used or new methods? Who collected the data; was this person independent? Is reliability and validity of the use tools addressed?
6	Methods	Methods for analysing data are sufficiently clear: Are methods for analysing qualitative data clearly described (who did the analysis, what is the role of this person, were accepted methods used and referred to)? Were exact statistical tests used to analyse quantitative data? Are confidence intervals, p values, measures of variation given where appropriate? If only a subset of all data is presented, is it clear how this was selected? Is it clear how incomplete data were dealt with?

7	Methods	Methods seem adequate to answer study question: Was an appropriate study design used to answer study question? Do the chosen methods provide sufficient valid data to answer the study questions? Is triangulation of methods and data used?
8	Methods/ Results	Any comparison that is done between groups is fair: Are the groups comparable with regard to baseline data? Are any differences here discussed? Is verified that any later differences in groups are only due to the IT intervention and not to external other factors such as staff changes?
9	Results	All results are credible and seem valid: Do the results give an answer to the initial research questions? Have the results been presented in a credible way? Is all data presented and interpreted? Are objective and subjective findings distinguished clearly?
10	Discussion (Conclusion)	All conclusions seem justified by the results: Have the results been well summarized? Have the results been well interpreted and reflected in the context of existing literature? Have the weaknesses of the study been mentioned? Is it made clear whether the results are transferable to other settings?

Figure 5. *Percentage of IT evaluation studies performed in single-unit, single-centered or multi-centered trials 1982-2005 (n=15 per 3-year period). The percentage selected studies from each time period is presented bracketed on the A-axis.*

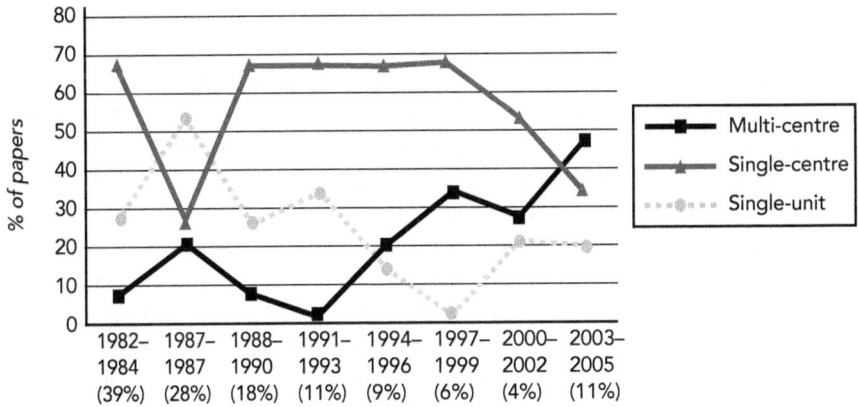

Conclusions

Finally, it should be noted that evaluation is an important part of developing and implementing an information system, especially when it concerns the major part of health space. The use of an evaluation framework is essential in order to all health information systems be assessed under the same light.

Therefore, the export of comparison results may not lead to any improvements or extensions to a system while we should not overlook the fact that each organization has its own peculiarities and special requirements. In other words, a MIS can be perfectly adapted, successfully implemented and have a strong acceptance by its users in a healthcare organization, while in another one to be failed.

In each evaluation model, the factors that are considered important are: people, technology and organization, and the degree coverage and their interaction are examined. The evaluation process shows similarities on how the data collection and analysis phases are, but we must not forget that it is a multifaceted process.

Ultimately, the need for better description of the collecting and analyzing data methods is necessary in studies designed to assess, although the quality of publications has improved over the last 24 years, providing a better understanding and knowledge of problems and abilities of a MIS.

YPAPANTI THERMOU is an undergraduate student at the University of Central Greece in the Department of Computer Science and Biomedical Informatics. Her scientific interests are in the area of Medical Information Systems and Electronic Health Records, including the implementation and evaluation of new technologies emphasizing in e-health aspects of administrative services.

YANNIS CHARALABIDIS is Assistant Professor in the University of Aegean, in the area of eGovernment Information Systems, while also heading eGovernment & eBusiness Research in the Decision Support Systems Laboratory of National Technical University of Athens (NTUA), planning and coordinating high-level policy making, research and pilot application projects for governments and enterprises worldwide. A computer engineer with a Ph.D. in complex information systems, he has been employed for eight years as an executive director in Singular IT Group, leading software development and company expansion in Eastern Europe. He writes and teaches on eGovernment Information Systems, Interoperability and Standardization, eParticipation and Government Transformation in NTUA and the University of Aegean.

ILIAS MAGLOGIANNIS received a diploma in Electrical & Computer Engineering and a Ph.D. in Biomedical Engineering and Medical Informatics from the National Technical University of Athens (NTUA) Greece in 1996 and 2000, respectively. He serves as Assistant Professor in the Department of Computer

Science and Biomedical Informatics in the University of Central Greece (www. dib.ucg.gr). He has been principal investigator in many European and National Research programs in Biomedical Engineering and Informatics. His scientific activities include biomedical informatics, image processing, multimedia and assistive technologies.

REFERENCES

Elske Ammenwerth, Stefan Graber, Gabriele Herrmann, Thomas Burkle, Jochem Konig, Evaluation of health information systems—problems and challenges, *International Journal of Medical Informatics* (2003) 71, 125-135, www.elsevier.com/locate/ijmedinf

Maryati Mohd. Yusof, Jasna Kuljis, Anastasia Papazafeiropoulou, Lampros K. Stergioulas, An evaluation framework for Health Information Systems: human, organization and technology-fit factors (HOT-fit), *International Journal of Medical Informatics* (2008) 77, 386-398, www.intl. elsevierhealth.com/journals/ijmi

Maryati Mohd. Yusof, Ray J. Paul, Lampros K. Stergioulas, Towards a Framework for Health Information Systems Evaluation, Proceedings of the 39th Hawaii International Conference on System sciences-2006, IEEE

N. F. De Keizer, E. Ammenwerth, The quality of evidence in health informatics: How did the quality of healthcare IT evaluation publications develop from 1982 to 005?, *International Journal of Medical Informatics* (2008) 77, 41-49, www.intl.elsevierhealth.com/journals/ijmi

Steven E. Labkoff, William A. Yasnoff, A framework for systematic evaluation of health information infrastructure progress in communities, *Journal of Medical Informatics* 40 (2007), 100-105, www.sciencedirect.com

Yung-Yu Su, John Fulcher, Khin Than Win, Herng-Chia Chiu, Cui-Fen Chiu, Evaluating the implementation of Electronic Medical Record (EMR) Systems from the perspective of Health Professional, 2008, IEEE 8th International Conference on Computer and Information Technology Workshops

Chapter 4

Main Tendencies and Prospects: ICT in Health

Patrice Cristofini, Alain Berard and Michel Daigne

Some general observations in 2008

Life expectancy at birth of the population increases. According to the National Institute for Demographic Studies (INED), about half of the French and European population will be over 50 years in 2050. Population ageing associated with the constantly increasing importance of the assumption of cost related to chronic diseases are key stakes of the Western health systems.

The impact of chronic diseases on our health system is very high as well as on the population as on the economy and financing. Long-term illness (LTI) concerns 7.7 million French, i.e. nearly 13% of the French population who at the same time consume 64% of the healthcare insurance expenditures—which represents average costs of 8,700 euros per patient. This number could reach 12 million insured persons in 2015.

A TEN-HMS study on patients with an increased risk of cardiac deficiency highlighted that remote monitoring leads to a reduction of 13% of the total costs of the assumption of responsibility of such pathologies. If we currently apply this modest assumption of a reduction of 10% for the LTI, we would get annual savings of 6.7 billion euros.

In parallel, the offer of healthcare services does not correspond to the needs of the population.

There are different possible explanations:

♦ epidemiological transition,
♦ insufficient replacement of the healthcare professionals going into retirement (shortage of healthcare professionals, unequal geographical repartition, remote regions…)

♦ no communication between the healthcare services in the city (self-employed activities), the healthcare services provided by hospitals and those provided by medico-social structures…

Information and Communication Technologies (ICT) can mitigate the effects of the shortage of professional resources (knowledge management, computerized digital files, tele-expertise, tele-diagnosis, remote support…), support the alternatives to traditional hospitalization and the development of home-based services, improve the quality of patient healthcare, as well as the effectiveness of the investments in health. They contribute to improve the access to the care, under better conditions and with lower costs.

Fifteen years from now, 25% of the French population will be concerned by ICT in the field of health. According to the Médiamétrie institute, more than 13.5 million households (50%) had access to the Internet during the first quarter of 2008 and more than 12.4 million had high speed Internet access (ADSL or cable). This should not hide the fact that the highest rates of Internet access were recorded in Iceland (84%), in the Netherlands (83%), in Sweden (79%) and in Denmark (78%) [Eurostat 2007]. French households spend approximately 115 euros per month on ICT; half of this is spent on cell phones.

An increasingly significant part of the French and European households (20% in 2015) will need products and services based on Information and Communication Technologies in particular to take care of their health. The Internet represents the main means of searching information on health for 65% of the French Net surfers.

Concerning the computerization of health professionals in France in 2007:

♦ 86% of the doctors are computerized; 19% of the general practitioners and 30% of the self-employed specialists do not have Internet at their work place (survey IPSOS Santé 2007). This rate is much weaker for the ancillary medical workers: 27% for the self-employed nurses and 15% for the self-employed physiotherapists.

♦ The hospital budget devoted to Information Systems amounts to 1.7% of the total expenditure of the health care institutions (3–4% in the USA). Within the framework of the "Plan Hospital 2012," this budget increase to 3%.

There is no comprehensive and global view of the requirements in ICT—hence the very complex environment, and the needs badly met or satisfied by expensive solutions offered by too few industrials[1]. Research or intervention programs (telemedicine or telehealth, general information on health…) are fragmented, without any links between each other, and are mainly determined by the technological challenges to meet. Research is not global but focused on an identified need related to a particular population group (disability, pathology). The financers are multiple and very variable corresponding to the technical systems and the type of vulnerability (handicap, seniority, pathology). They are facing a very fragmented and sometimes redundant market. This situation does not enable economies of scale and products or services are not provided at an industrial scale.

Industrials ask for clear rules concerning market access, the efficient size of these markets and the development potentialities. The financing of these markets is mainly public, even if the private sector is involved, and the commercial marketing strategies are often ineffective. The rules for evaluation and the criteria for acceptance of the ICT projects launched in the area of health are not public or put in place …

The ICT

ICT facilitate the access to and the sharing of information but should not be reduced to a simple computer or information system. These two systems represent the basis for ICT. ICT also make it possible to overcome certain handicaps (via home automation for example) and/or to renew a social link (videoconference, video-discussion…).

After several years of developing telehealth for professionals (telemedicine), ICT are now used for the development of the entire spectrum of personalized health (p-health) for the patients and the public. ICT for health is related to telemedecine, "Web-health" as well as p-health.

Telemedicine is the realization of a medical act performed at distance via the use of ICT tools.

Telemedicine covers four activities:

♦ Teleconsultation: a medical act carried out in the presence of the patient who dialogues with the consulted doctor (cancerology, psychiatry, penitentiary medicine…)

♦ Tele-expertise (including tele-diagnosis): any act of diagnosis and/or therapeutic act which is carried out between two doctors and outside of the presence of the patient (perinatality, nephrovigilance, tele-imagery, or tele-radiology, rare diseases…)

♦ Remote monitoring: a medical act which results from the transmission (telemetry) and the interpretation of clinical, radiological or biological data by a doctor, collected by the patient (himself or via a device) or by a health professional. It is the case for monitoring of arterial hypertension/

cardiac failure, the follow-up of coagulation drugs , fetal tele-monitoring, hemodialysis, retinography…)

♦ Remote support: a doctor assists remotely another health professional carrying out a medical or surgical act, an act of care, radiology…

It should be mentioned that in the DHOS report "The place of telemedicine in the organization of care" of November 2008, neither tele-training nor the geo-localization (via GPS) were considered as an activity of telemedicine.

Web-health includes the totality of Internet resources usable by the patient (or his family) or by the professional, including Personal Medical Records (PMR).

The French legislation (Public Health Code) forbids drug trade (armchair shopping) and the realization of medical acts for a patient (except telemedicine). Web-health includes three types of sites:

♦ Sites providing informative content (databases, forum…): e.g. "doctissimo" which is a medical site for the general public including articles, discussion forums, chats and blogs.

♦ Promotional sites: e-Trade (drugstores for parapharmaceutical needs, dietetics, fitness, complement proteins…)

♦ Transaction processing sites via applicative solutions: such sites require subscription (subject to a charge) and provide access to files/downloadable tools or health applications, and also allow exchanges between its members. Example sites are the online employment offer in EHPAD[2] (French establishments providing care for the dependent *elderly*; e.g. homes for the elderly), allowing to download software calculating the level of dependence of elderly persons ("girage"), the balanced average GIR (the "weight" of the dependent residents in a EHPAD).

Due to the diffusion of mobile telephony and geo-localization devices the concept of p-health is developing. p-Health is a northern American concept. In a context of the development of chronic diseases, the patient who lives with his disease becomes the expert just as well as the doctor and even more. The patient is the person in charge of but also the decision maker concerning his care. For this reason, he must have access to all related information (access to the Electronic Medical Record).

Tendencies

The economic impact of ICT is increasing: ICT represent today approximately 2.5 billion euros, that is to say 1.5% of the health expenditure. According to European studies, this percentage will reach 5% within the five next years.

Corresponding to the EITO (European Information Technology Observatory), the domain of Information and Communication Technologies attained a growth of 3.5% within the European Union in 2007.

The Institute for Prospective Technology Studies reminds us that the pensioners of tomorrow are the today 50-years-olds, but about half of them has a cell phone and more than the third has a computer at home. Strengthening the use of ICT by seniors should further enrich the demand of new media based services. This would contribute to reduce the phenomenon of the "fearful"[3] described by the Americans.

In the context of information services, the development of multi-channel and multi-port services represents an important contribution both for the health sector as for the rest of the Information Society. The new protocols should in particular allow a wide accessibility of health related information. The development of audio contents should for example facilitate the access of the partially-sighted persons to this information.

The administrative services, and in particular the computerized medical files, could also benefit from new technological developments. The evolution of ICT towards an increased mobility of the users should enable the health professionals to use ICT tools more effectively. Additionally, standardization should increase the interoperability of the systems. And last but not least, the estimated evolution in the area of smart cards should allow a significant improvement of secured administrative health services. Example: a self-employed nurse is filling in a data sheet relating to a patient's care, capillary blood glucose etc. on a PDA at the home of the diabetic patient. The data are immediately transmitted to a health network for diabetology.

Telemedicine

The aptitude and the will of the patients to take charge of their health is increasing. It will become necessary to recognize the remote medical acts and to refund them, especially in view of the coming shortage healthcare professionals.

The non-refunding of remote medical acts in France penalizes the French market. All the more as a growing number of European countries (Germany, Portugal, Netherlands, the United Kingdom…) evolve towards the recognition of this type of acts and their financing (Germany since January 1, 2008 for cardiology).

The most innovative developments of ICT tools specific to the healthcare sector should concern tele-health. Indeed, technologies enabling remote monitoring or tele-expertise should considerably evolve, in particular in order to compensate the (quantitative and qualitative) lack of healthcare professionals and to make it possible in certain cases to ensure a constancy of care.

Tele-assistance and the development of "smart homes" should thus facilitate home care of dependent people (home automation). Positioning and localization tools (via Galileo or GPS) can increase the mobility of the users and facilitate the provision of emergency services, or the monitoring of high-risk patients (Alzheimer, insufficient chronic respiratory …) without giving the feeling of being under surveillance.

The medical imagery will also develop, what constitutes an essential precondition for the development of tele-surgery or tele-treatment.

All this requires a much more developed hospital information system, real interoperability of the systems, secured email and broadband, and a telemedicine coupled with education and training for operational health…

Web-health

Over the last decade, the consultation of Internet sites devoted to healthcare exploded. Nearly 10 million Net surfers visited a website related to healthcare or well-being in April 2008 (33% of the Net surfers), which represents an increase of 53% between April 2007 and 2008 (source: Médiamétrie). Médiamétrie states that in April, 33.2 million Net surfers over 11 years were connected to the Internet. This represents an increase of 14% in one year; 27 million of them have high speed Internet at home.

People mainly seek information and explanations concerning a symptom, a pathology or a treatment but also wish to get into contact with other patients or families having the same health problems in order to share experiences, advices and "tricks" (discussion forum). This phenomenon modifies the relation between the people cared for and the health professionals.

The use of Internet completely changes relations and the phenomenon of information asymmetry. Certain professionals already understood these expectations and created websites with a high informational and educational value. Associations of patients, users and/or families followed these examples (Association Alzheimer France, CISS Inter-Association Health Collective …). These websites provide medical, legal, and social information. People can download information folders, communication and evaluation tools.

Consumers' associations and associations of patients and former patients want to hold a central place in the dissemination of information. On Internet sites, they exchange their experiences, share information, propose discussion forums, and encourage the creation of blogs and other initiatives (social networking).

This expresses an important need for information, but it is also the will of the patients and their families, by becoming indispensable, to participate in taking the decisions they are affected by (p-health).

As far as technology is concerned, the new demand for equipment and information systems in the field of healthcare is characterized by some important tendencies:

♦ a miniaturization and a geographical dispersion of the medical devices that are now communicating with each other and likely to be implanted in the human body (nano-medicine). In this regard, industries worldwide are progressing very fast and future developments will probably depend more on the ethical, sociological and economic concerns than on technical constraints;

♦ an increased performance and complexity of the technical platforms of the hospitals, which are increasingly communicating (between each others and with the city);

♦ an increasing inter-connectivity of the information systems – between each other but also with biological measurement and observation devices as well as with dedicated terminals entrusted to the patients;

♦ a trend towards generalized interconnection of the organizations, offices, laboratories, and domestic equipment;

♦ a foreseeable development of telehealth and the facilities enabling home care and social rehabilitation (videoconference, vocal device...)

PATRICE CRISTOFINI has worked since November 2007 as Head of Strategic Alliances and Partnerships of the Orange Healthcare Division. He served before successively as Head of Healthcare at the national and international level with major international corporations, including Sema Group (2000), Schlumberger (2002) and Atos Origin (2004) for occupational health and strategic development of the e-healthcare offering for the general management. He is a member of the Institut Montaigne's healthcare "think tank," CEPS institute (non governmental organization affiliated to european council) and adviser to the Mederic Group in the field of prevention. He is also Honorary President and current President of AFTIM (French Association of Technicians, Engineers and Occupational Health physicians). He is also Director of the quarterly publication "Sécurité et Médecine du Travail" (Safety and Occupational Medicine) and co-author of "Médecine du Travail et Santé Publique: quel avenir ?" ("Occupational Medicine and Public Health: What Future?") published by Editions de Santé.

ALAIN BÉRARD is a medical doctor (public health specialist) and a health economist. After a hospital and university career, he now manages a big health network (viral infections, addictions, diabetes, old persons, cancer) in Paris, France. He works on health and social policies, and their evaluation. So he needs data from hospital information systems and follows with interest the evolution of information and communication technology (ICT). He published several articles on health policies and their evaluation. The last works concerned the costs of building of a national health program in France, and the economic impact of not quality in company on the general economy, as well.

MICHEL DAIGNE is Professor of engineering of the Health of the Ecole Centrale Paris and Director of ISAM Resources. He steered during the 1970s a department of research in France of the American company Burroughs, where he acquired a first experience of the economic and social world. In the 1980s, he ruled the department anesthetize, resuscitation, surgery and implantable devices of the National Center of the Hospital Equipment in France. In the 1990s, he created the company of engineering and consulting of the health ISAM Ressources, co-based Centrale Santé, and he is Professor of engineering of the Health of the Ecole Centrale Paris today, where he is in charge of the master's degree "Management and Technology of establishments and networks of Health" and where he animates the development of the executive training in health and biotechnologies. He accompanies at the same time several projects of organization in health concerning establishments of various regions and areas of medical specialization. And the perinatal health, the respiratory health, the health in the work and the gerontology are the priority domains of its theoretical and practical activities. He formalized a first experience of these organizations in the book "Reform the Health by Networks" published in the Editions de la Santé with a group of doctors of public health.

ENDNOTES

1. Report "Usage des TIC par les patients et les citoyens en situation de fragilité dans leurs lieux de vie"

2. EHPAD: établissement hébergeant des personnes âgées dépendantes

3. Unfounded fear or lack of confidence of the elderly regarding technology

References

Pierre Simon & Dominique Acker: Rapport DHOS "La place de la télémédecine dans l'organisation des soins," November 2008

Confidential note of the Ministry of Economy, Finances and Industry (Bercy), September 2008

Robert Picard: Rapport "Enjeux des TIC pour l'aide à l'autonomie des patients et des citoyens en situation de handicap ou de fragilité dans leurs lieux de vie," May 2008

Claudette Humbert-Mulas & Robert Picard: Report "Télémédecine et accès au marché," February 2008

Bernhard Rohleder: Tendances du marché des TIC en Europe et en France, BITKOM, November 2007

Executive summary "Une filière des équipements et TIC de santé au service de l'intérêt national," SNITEM—LESISS, 2007

Robert Picard: Report "TIC et santé: quelle politique publique?," August 2007

Robert Picard: Report "Usage des TIC par les patients et les citoyens en situation de fragilité dans leurs lieux de vie," August 2007

Vincent Rialle: Report "Technologies nouvelles susceptibles d'améliorer les pratiques gérontologiques et la vie quotidienne des malades âgés et de leur famille," May 2007

Maurice Levy & Jean-Pierre Jouyet: "L'économie de l'immatériel: la croissance de demain," Ministry of Economy, Finances and Industry, November 2006

Observatoire de l'intranet, Report 2004.

Chapter 5

Asthma and SARS Grid— An Introduction to the Use of Medical Grid-based Applications in Taiwan

Shu-Hui (Bonita) Hung

In today's modern healthcare environment, medical care is largely supported by high technology equipment and devices such as the Internet and advanced wireless technologies. Informatics Technology Communication (ITC) platforms help physicians provide high quality, long-term healthcare services to their patients both at home and in the hospital.

The Medical Grid-based platform described in this study utilizes advanced networking technologies and consumer mobile phones to develop a communication channel between the patient and physician when the patient is at the hospital and/or at home. In particular, the advanced capabilities of today's modern Internet-enabled mobile phones provide the patient with convenient access to their health-related information both at home and in the hospital. This service has been successfully implemented and extensively tested both overseas and here in Taiwan.

This study demonstrates that the ITC platform provides valuable experience and optimal results in the long-term care of chronic (e.g. asthma) and epidemic (e.g. SARS) diseases.

Asthma Grid (Year 2003–2008)

The main idea behind Asthma Grid is to focus on improving the quality of the patient's home-based healthcare service. This includes self-education on how to live with and treat asthma, the long-term recording of the patient's *peak expiratory flow* (PEFR) *measurement*, and providing a service that allows the patient to self-monitor changes in his symptoms.

The platform includes a real-time assessment/response feature that is particularly useful. Once a patient submits his data to the server via his mobile phone, the short message service (SMS) automatically sends an assessment report back to the patient's mobile phone alerting him of information relevant to his current asthma condition and sending him, for example, weather-related precautionary "warning" messages (e.g. high local pollen count that might adversely affect his asthma condition).

Asthma Grid also includes an around-the-clock auto-monitoring and alert system to assist both the patient and physician when the patient's medical condition changes drastically. Also, the Asthma Grid-enabled mobile phone offers the asthma patient pertinent and up-to-date weather-related information so that the patient can take extra precautions when, for example, there is an extremely high pollen count that might have a very negative effect on this asthma symptoms. Asthma Grid also incorporates a feature called the Location-Based System (LBS) that provides physicians and rescue teams the exact location of the patient in case of emergency.

Background

More than 1,000,000 people in Taiwan suffer from asthma, and it is responsible for 1,200+ deaths annually. Also, according to Taiwan's official government statistics on asthma, more than one-third of the 1,000,000 cases are categorized as "severe" or "possibly life threatening." These patients classified as "severe" are often in and out of the hospital frequently because of their asthma. If they must receive in-patient care in the hospital, the high cost is borne by the National Healthcare System and, ultimately, the Taiwanese tax payers. If these emergency room and in-patient visits could be avoided, the cost savings would be tremendous.

According to government statistics, the great majority of individuals who die from asthma in Taiwan are the middle-aged primary wage earners of their family. These deaths are true tragedies and a great loss not only to the families but also to the society and the country as a whole. Also, according to government statistics, 6%–10% of Taiwan's total healthcare budget is spent on treating asthma patients. With proper care and treatment, asthma normally does not kill and, in fact, most patients can go on living normal lives.

Many asthma patients in Taiwan regularly travel around the island for business or study. Sometimes the local weather conditions such as dust storms may trigger an asthmatic attack. Thus, the platform integrates real-time weather reports in order to inform the patience of such conditions, and, as a result, prevent an asthmatic attack from occurring.

The Taiwanese government has designed a program that utilizes specially developed measurement procedures to encourage physicians to closely examine their asthma patients over a 12-month period and then record/input their patient's data. The primary goal of this program is to study ways in which to treat asthma patients on an out-patient basis and, thus, reduce the medical cost associated with asthma care and, at the same time, improve the quality of living among asthma patients.

The emphasis of the program is on collecting the patients' clinical data on-site as well as encouraging the asthma patients to upload their healthcare-related data from home everyday using their mobile phone. As an incentive for the physicians and their patients to participate in the program, the Taiwanese government offers annual incentive bonuses to those physicians who successfully complete the year-long program. This policy provides a good incentive for physicians to encourage their asthma patients to participate in the program.

In order for the physicians to receive their incentive bonuses, they must successfully establish a multi-stage home-based clinical database for their asthma patients that includes the patient's daily medicine dosage, daily activities, and self-education development. Each stage requires the physician to monitor the patient's "checkpoints" which are established by governmental policy. In the past, the physician would usually assign one of his staff members to do the required paperwork and make the necessary phone calls, however, using the modern technologies provided by Asthma Grid, this is no longer necessary. By using the platform's integrated tools, the physician can easily and quickly perform the online work himself taking advantage of this value-added service. This service fully meets the needs not only of the physicians, but also the local government and patients as well.

Objectives
The main objectives of this study are:

♦ To eliminate the extra man-power needed to provide the service, cut the cost of asthma care service, and improve the overall effectiveness of the asthma healthcare service.

♦ To improve the asthma patient's quality of living by developing the mobile phone's Internet-based functions so that they better meet the patient's needs.

Technologies Design
The service has been divided into three distinct modes as a result of the input from various users: 1) web-based, 2) home phone-based, and 3) mobile phone-based modes/services. The web-based service allows both physicians and patients to input clinic data into the asthma patient's database using a common personal computer (PC). With the web-based service, patients are encouraged

to key their data into the website on a daily basis. This results in a daily report being generated to the physician specific to each individual patient.

The focus of the home phone-based mode is on enabling elderly patients who do not know how to use a PC to participate in the Asthma Grid program. Instead of using a PC, elderly patients are able to input their data using an ordinary home telephone (i.e. landline) via a voice response unit (VRU) that is made up of easy-to-follow audible instructions. After the elderly patient has input his data using his home phone, the platform automatically generates an assessment message for the patient. In response to requests from users for additional mobility, user-friendly access, and safety and security issues, the mobile phone phase was recently developed and is currently in use.

These three different "modes" provide both physicians and patients a well-organized service that takes into consideration the various physical locations of the patient. Between the three phases, the mobile phone service has received the most widespread use (Fig. 1).

Fig. 1. *Asthma Care via Mobile Phone flowchart*

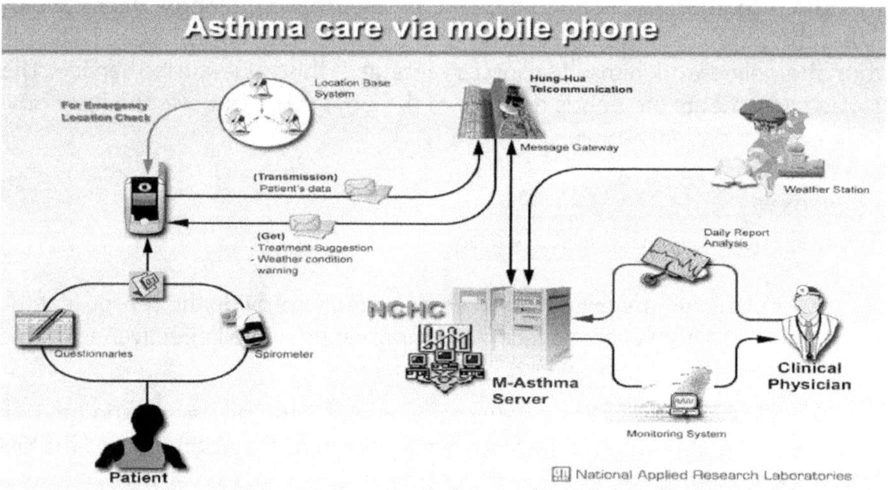

The Asthma Grid web-based platform allows physicians to easily manage and maintain their list of asthma patients. It also allows them to provide better and more timely healthcare to their patients by allowing them to access their patient's data online anytime and anywhere. In that the patient's data is input according to the standards set by Taiwan's National Healthcare System, the physicians are also able to use the system to easily and quickly upload their patient's data to the government's asthma statistical information database. Once the data has been uploaded and verified, the physician is then automatically notified of its acceptance by the government database management team. If the asthma patient's status indicates that he was well cared for over the program's a one year period, the physician is eligible for the incentive bonus.

The mobile phone mode of the Asthma Grid platform provides the greatest mobility for both the physician and the asthma patient. The "smart phone" is used as the mobile device for the mobile phone mode because its operating system and environment supports Java/Java scripts (Fig. 2).

The infrastructure of the Asthma Grid mobile phone mode is based on the Java/Java EE platform. The mobile phone mode infrastructure includes the asthma patient care system, environment data collecting system, patient case record system, and mobile phone interface. The mobile phone interface integrates with the general packet radio service (GPRS). The remainder of the system functions are based on the web browser. (Fig. 3).

Fig. 2. Mobile phone PEFR input interface

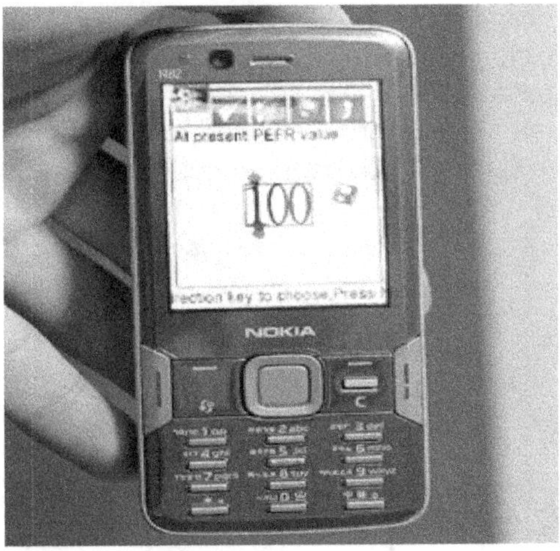

Fig. 3. Asthma Grid infrastructure

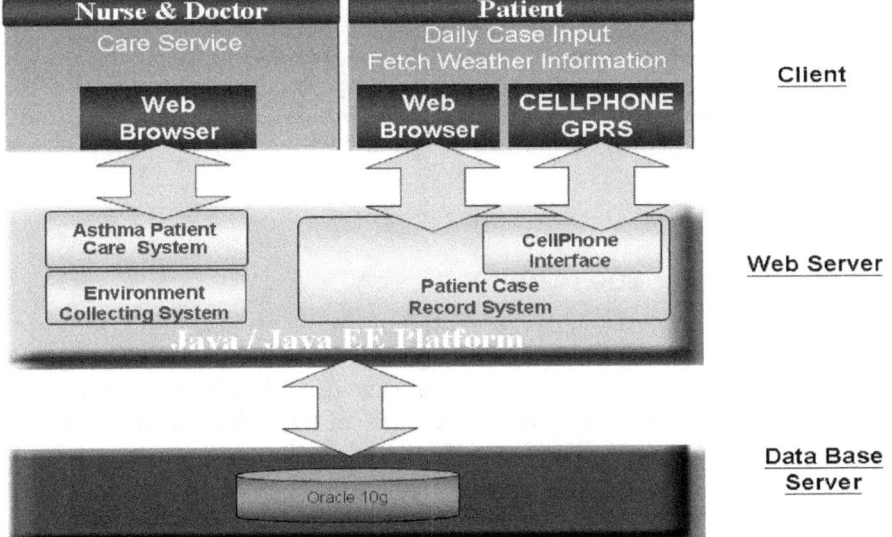

Results

This Asthma Grid platform is designed to meet the needs of the government, the physician, and the patient. These needs include the reduction of hospitalization expenses, providing an efficient method to assist physicians in the management of their asthma patients, and to offer a superior service to the asthma patients directly. This program is slated to run for a term of five years.

According to the Northern Regional Branch of the Bureau of National Health Insurance, the Asthma Grid platform was utilized by a total of 384 clinics and hospitals 2002–2005. A total of 13,399 patients who were considered "severe" asthma cases joined this study as compared with 34,585 asthma patients that received "traditional" care for their "less-severe" asthma symptoms. The Asthma Grid program resulted in an estimated total savings of NT 160,778,000 (USD $4,729,000) for the period 2002–2005. (Fig.4)

Fig. 4. *The result of asthma grid*

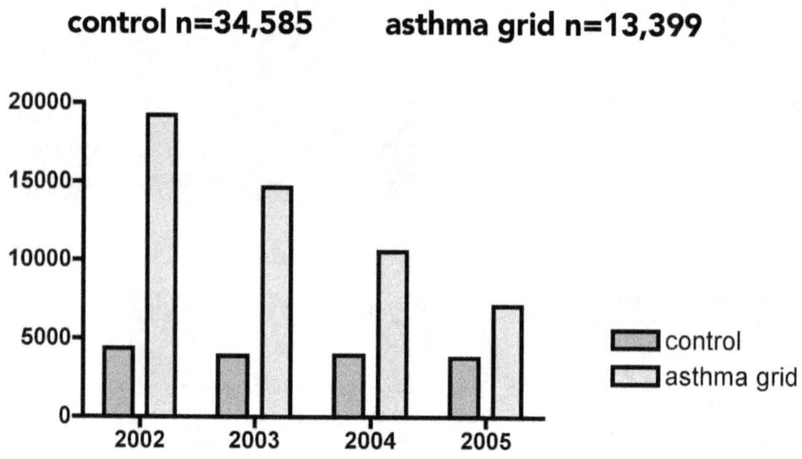

SARS Grid (Year 2003–2005)

SARS Grid was successfully implemented in two Taiwanese SARS-dedicated hospitals and two medical centers during the 2003 worldwide SARS outbreak. SARS Grid's two most noteworthy benefits were 1) it utilized technology to help control the panic caused by the outbreak of the SARS epidemic (i.e. During the SARS outbreak, there were some individuals who developed SARS-like symptoms who committed suicide due to the stigma associated with having SARS) and 2) to provide a virtual environment for physicians to gain control over the disease both inside and outside of local hospitals and clinics and to understand the patient's historical data before providing treatment.

The SARS Access Grid-based video teleconferencing system (VTC) allowed physicians to collect, organize, and share SARS patients' medical records among other (oft times quarantined) physicians, clinics, and hospitals. SARS Grid also served as an effective means by which to assist in the physical transferring of SARS patients (and their medical data) from one hospital/clinic to another. Also, SARS Grid served as a go-between between home-isolated and/or quarantined SARS patients and their hospitals, clinics, and physicians.

The SARS Grid platform successfully demonstrated that such web-based informatics tools can be used to significantly increase public awareness of diseases such as SARS. SARS Grid was also used to help gain control over the SARS outbreak in Taiwan and effectively reduce the number of infections in local area hospitals and clinics. The SARS Grid platform concept has great potential for use again in case of future similar epidemic disease outbreaks.

Background

In April 2003, the entire world's population began to recognize that it was facing a real threat to the public health. In early 2003, Severe Acute Respiratory Syndrome (SARS) spread rapidly and seemingly uncontrollably across Asia and to the North American continent. As more and more cases of this new and life threatening disease popped up in the news, a panic began to set in. The sheer speed at which the SARS outbreak was spreading greatly alarmed the world's top medical experts. There simply was no historical information on which to begin looking for a cure for this disease. The panic over the SARS outbreak became so intense in Taiwan that, by the end of April 2003, the federal government made the difficult decision to quarantine about 100 staff and patients at a local area hospital. The entire hospital, located in Taipei, was quarantined due to an unusually high incidence of the hospital's staff and patients coming down with SARS-like symptoms. The Department of Public Health, Taipei City Government made the decision to try to bring back all the visitors who had visited the hospital for the two weeks prior and test them for the SARS virus. Unfortunately, the people who had visited the local hospital were extremely reluctant to return for testing because they feared they would also be quarantined.

It was later documented that some of the people who had visited the hospital had, in fact, contracted the SARS virus while visiting the hospital but did not return to the hospital for testing, treatment, and quarantine. Due to this unfortunate situation, a second wave of the SARS infections hit Taiwan's general population. This second wave was believed to have been further spread via the public transportation system, physical contact between infected victims and their family members, and many medical experts. Many of the victims of the second wave of the SARS epidemic also had to be hospitalized. This put a tremendous strain on the already extremely overburdened area hospitals.

Objectives

♦ To educate and provide accurate information regarding SARS to the general public,

♦ To provide effective monitoring of suspected SARS-infected patients whom were home-bound,

♦ To provide a virtual VTC room for medical experts to discuss their SARS cases and share diagnosis and methods of treatment in order to help reduce the spread of the infection,

♦ To establish a digital data transferring service between hospitals and clinics, thus, helping to reduce the spread of the virus,

♦ To provide real-time statistical references and data to governmental decision-makers.

Technology Design

The SARS Grid prototype application provides for distributed VTC, case study and discussion, and is suitable for installation and implementation within the hospital environment. The SARS Grid platform allows for the running of multiple participants and discussion rooms simultaneously. Each participant can simultaneously view all other participants and conference rooms within a single window/interface.

The SARSHope website was designed to help contain the spread of the SARS virus by providing public education, patient diagnosis and treatment, monitoring, and management of the disease. For the home-bound SARS patient, the SARSHope website also helped provide residential isolation control and included a body temperature monitoring function. If the home-bound SARS patient were to input data indicating that his health condition was worsening, his local health center would then automatically receive an alert requiring immediate patient follow up. The local health center could then arrange for, if necessary, an ambulance to pick up and transfer the patient to a hospital for treatment.

The SARSHope website also incorporated a function that alerted the patient's doctor while, at the same time, sending the patient's detailed medical history to the clinic/hospital. If the doctor needed additional assistance diagnosing the case, he could easily call a meeting with other doctors from other hospitals using SARS Grid's Access Grid-based VTC feature (Fig.5).

Fig. 5. *SARS Grid medical data sharing function*

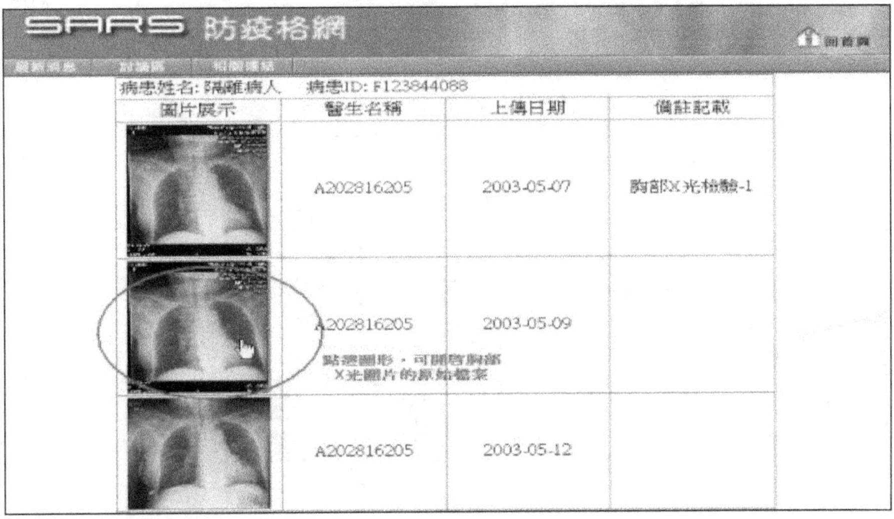

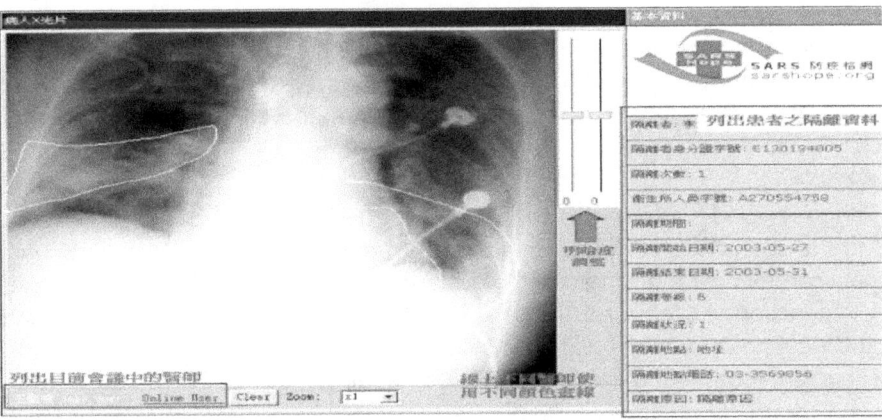

The SARS Grid platform included a whiteboard function that allowed physicians in different hospitals to gather virtually to discuss suspected cases and treatment methods, share patient data, etc. (Fig. 6).

Fig. 6. *The SARS Grid whiteboard function allowed physicians to share patient information and data*

The local health centers were able to use the SARSHope website to help control quarantined rooms and to update the patient's medical information. Based on the information submitted by the local health centers, the areas where the highest outbreak of the SARS virus had been detected could be easily identified and avoided (Fig. 6). During the SARS outbreak, the NCHC setup seven Access Grid nodes at local health centers, medical centers, and SARS-dedicated hospitals (Fig. 7).

Fig. 7. *The SARS Grid flowchart*

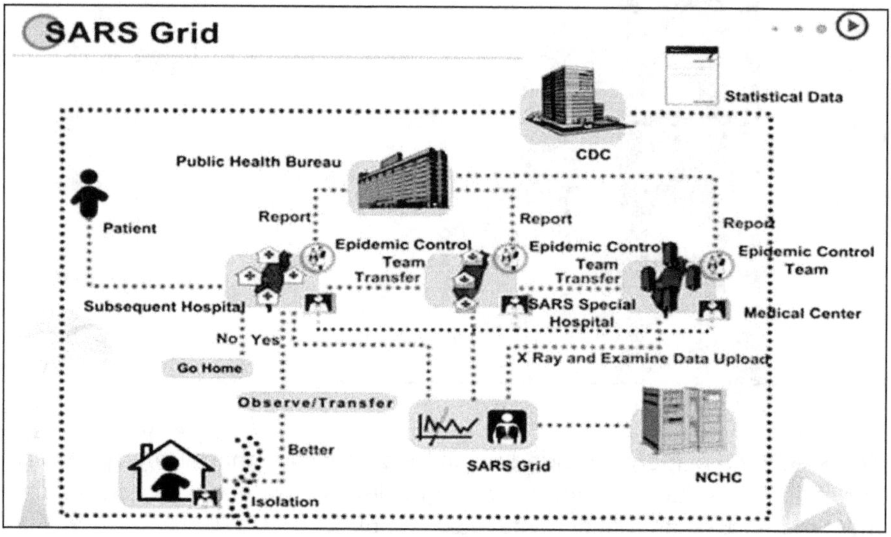

The SARSHope web site included the patient's personal information, his ten day contact history (i.e. the individuals the patient had come in contact with over the past ten days), and medical information, including medical images. The SARSHope website also contained many management functions to help minimize the spread of the SARS virus. These functions included the number of suspected and confirmed SARS cases, the number of rooms in hospitals and clinics that were quarantined, and the number of home-bound SARS victims.

Results

The SARS Grid platform was successfully used to 1) educate the public regarding the spread of the SARS virus and 2) to help Taiwan's medical community gain control over the spread of the disease. In particular, the Access Grid-based VTC function of SARS Grid allowed physicians to share and transfer patient data and treatment methods without having to physically move from one hospital/clinic to the other and, in so doing, risk spreading the virus even further.

The SARSHope website allowed the general public to register online and input/record their body temperature as well as instruct them on how to perform a self-examination for SARS-related symptoms. Also, the SARSHope website provided information regarding additional resources should the user have questions about SARS or need more information.

During the SARS epidemic in Taiwan, individuals suspected of contracting the SARS virus were ordered by the National Healthcare System officials to stay in home isolation for a period of 7–10 days. During that period, those individuals used the SARS Grid platform to input their data so that local health experts could monitor their health condition. More than 10,000 individuals were registered on the SARSHope website during the duration of the SARS epidemic.

In the hospital setting, SARS Grid provided physicians with extremely useful features and tools including VTC, whiteboard, and patient data sharing and transferring capabilities. In Taiwan, there were three medical centers, two SARS-dedicated hospitals, and four off-shore health centers that joined the SARS Grid program.

Conclusions

This study illustrates that information technology can provide an effective and efficient methodology to traditional business models and services. It is important to realize that, no matter how IT is used to increase the effectiveness of a business/service model, there will always be the need to address the human side as well. The key to success then becomes how to win your customer's heart and trust.

Through this study, we discovered that the key to a successful business model is to provide a "total solution" to the customer that thoughtfully addresses each of his needs. Additionally, we found that effective communication between different users and developers is also key to the model's success.

SHU-HUI (BONITA) HUNG received her B.S. degree in Information Engineering from Eastern Washington University, Washington, U.S.A. in 1993. She received her M.S. degree in Mathematic and Computer Science Education from Oregon State University, Oregon, U.S.A. in 1997. Hung was interested in e-learning or media education through the deployment and execution of business information system, medical and healthcare informatics, with hands-on training courses teaching experiences and so on. Since 2002, she has been an associate researcher in Department of Bio & Medical Information Science, National Center for High-performance Computing, Taiwan, R.O.C. Her work experience is more approaching to integrate the new technologies in order to provide innovative medical or health care services to physicians and patients in these days. Hung has been practical executed few medical care projects completely and successfully in Taiwan. She now is currently working toward her Ph.D. degree in Department of Engineering Science, National Cheng Kung University, Taiwan, R.O.C. Hung's research interests include medical/health information and wireless transmission.

References

WHO "Severe Acute Respiratory Syndrome (SARS)" http://www.who.int/csr/sars/en/

American CDC http://www.cdc.gov/

http://www.cdc.gov/ncidod/sars/cht/index.htm

Health Canada http://www.hcsc.gc.ca/english/protection/warnings/sars/

Singapore Ministry of Health http://www.gov.sg/moh/sars/index.html

Hong Kong Department of Health http://www.info.gov.hk/dh/ap.htm

http://www.ssm.gov.mo/design/news/c_cdc_news.htm

http://www.doh.gov.tw/newverprog/proclaim/sars_list.asp

http://www.cdc.gov.tw/sars/

Acknowledgments

1. Chang-Gung Medical Foundation. Dr. Han-Pin Kuo, Taiwan

2. Argonne National Laboratory, Chicago, U.S.

Chapter 6

Extending the Horizon of eHealth

Ilias Iakovidis[1], European Commission, DG Information Society and Media, ICT for Health

Introduction

A healthy population and an innovation-friendly, sustainable economy are indispensable prerequisites for a wealthy society. Europe is currently going through a major demographic change that will affect both the economy and healthcare systems. One of the direct consequences will be the increased prevalence of chronic diseases, leading not only to a higher number of people with reduced independence and quality of life, but also to productivity loss due to prolonged absence or reduced capacity of the workforce. As an example, cardiovascular diseases alone are responsible for 42% of all deaths in the EU, 21% of productivity losses and costs to the EU economy of €192 billion a year. In the case of diabetes, more than 190 million patients worldwide need to be cared for, and in countries like Finland, the annual cost of managing a diabetic patient with complications exceeds €8.000. Chronic diseases are now responsible for the consumption of the vast majority of healthcare resources—more than 70% in developed countries—and are inflicting a transition in healthcare practice from acute to chronic care.

As a market, health and wellness comprises a total of up to 25% of the economy at large (when measured in employment, expenditure and value added), making it the largest industry of our economy and giving millions of households their vocational and financial basis. It is commonly understood that today's way of working and the existing structures of European healthcare systems have been exhausting human and financial resources. Supported by a large research community and by experts on medical technologies, most health authorities are planning national or regional reforms. Reform efforts focus on two fields of action: improving the productivity and cost effectiveness of existing healthcare systems; and transforming the existing structures and responsibilities of all stakeholders to develop new ways of health delivery and patient engagement. In both domains, Information and Communication Technologies (ICT) will play a crucial role. Moreover, the horizon of eHealth needs to be extended beyond merely healthcare. The utilisation of ICT can contribute to our understanding of all three determinants that impact on human health and their interrelationships: the healthcare system, nature, and nurture.

Beyond the current scope and definition of eHealth

For several decades, the traditional aim of eHealth has been the improvement of quality and productivity in healthcare. So far, the benefits from eHealth such as access, quality, and efficiency have been proven on a small scale only. A more rigorous assessment of eHealth benefits on a large scale (multi-center, regional or national scales, with participation of hundreds of health professionals and/or thousands of patients) has not yet become common place. This is partially due to the expense involved and the difficulty of applying existing and widely accepted methods such as randomised clinical trials.

However, a number of integrated, regional health information systems and networks—for instance in Spain, Italy, France and Sweden—have undergone a thorough socio-economic assessment. Those systems proved to be beneficial to a number of stakeholders involved—patients and their carers, health professional teams, health provider organisations and health authorities, thus enhancing the access to as well as the quality and efficiency of healthcare.[2] For example, an analysis of the regional health information system of the public health service in Andalusia showed total net benefits (i.e. overall socio-economic benefits minus overall costs) of 490 million EUR from the first year of planning in 1999 to 2010.[3]

Currently, many publications embroider enormous promises and potential based on projections of benefits from small-size pilots. Yet such claims can have the opposite effect on long term support and large scale deployments. The Directorate General *Information Society and Media* (DG INFSO) of the European Commission is presently supporting such large scale efforts through the *Competitiveness and Innovation Programme* (CIP) and studies on assessment methodologies for eHealth services.

A larger target for eHealth emerged during the nineties: ICT-enabled, patient-centred health systems that facilitate shared care and continuity of care through collaboration among health professionals. Over the last 15 years, DG INFSO has supported hundreds of research and demonstration projects in this domain. The kernel of these efforts was the development of interoperable electronic health record systems providing, at the point of need, timely and secure vital patient data to health professionals.[4]

Today, we are ready to enlarge the scope of eHealth even further, beyond healthcare, to consider all factors impacting human health. The central argument of this paper is that ICT is essential for understanding the entire picture of the health status of an individual or a population. ICT enhances a fully integrative approach to health by enabling progress in each of the three major health determinants:

- ♦ **Healthcare**—access, quality and efficiency of healthcare delivery
- ♦ **Nature**—or endogenous determinants (e.g. genetic predispositions)
- ♦ **Nurture**—or exogenous determinants (e.g. nutrition, lifestyle, environment).

There is limited knowledge about the determinants of health, their interplay and how to improve them. For example, it is known that only 10% of the factors contributing to premature death relate to healthcare while 40% relate to behavioural patterns, 30% to genetic predisposition, 15% to social circumstances and 5% to environmental factors.[5] This is not reflected in today's health service provision at all.

Only when we master these determinants will we be able to implement and fully realise the aspired shifts from care to prevention and from treatment to cure and healing. In this ambitious understanding of eHealth, we need to foster interdisciplinary research and bring two currently underutilised resources into play: information and patients. ICT is a well-suited tool to generate value from unused, scattered, complex or otherwise inaccessible information. ICT can also substantially contribute to the empowerment of patients/consumers through the provision of relevant information, health status monitoring and management, and support to lifestyle choices.

ICT for Healthcare Delivery

As outlined above, the main focus of eHealth has historically been on improved quality and efficiency of healthcare delivery systems—to build connectivity and digitisation. Today, Europe is leading the world in terms of connectivity among health organisations and ICT use in primary care[6]. This provides great possibilities for further productivity gains[7] and increased quality and safety of healthcare. Fully connecting public health authorities, researchers and clinicians to improve communication flow will help create *situational awareness* enabling the prediction and timely response to public health events such as SARS, avian flu, H1N1. Such a high level of connectivity and digitisation lays a much-needed foundation for bringing patients on board, and for better understanding and managing the two other factors influencing our health: nature and nurture.

ICT for Nature

In the area of nature, ICT has been a driving force behind new research in biology and projects such as the Human Genome Project. *Google Body*-like capabilities to visualise the human body and its functions from sub-cellular to organ levels can foster the development of personalised medicine, make medical interventions and surgery safer, and support medical research. The effort of translating the genetic make-up of an individual (or population) to the corresponding health risks and personalised medicine is a long-term project. Success will depend on bringing together, on a large scale, health information from both biological and clinical research combined with data from daily patient care, in full respect of privacy and confidentiality. To realise the full potential of research on healthcare and health (biological and environmental) data, large infrastructural developments at EU scale are needed as well as tools to process, visualise and communicate information and knowledge.

ICT for Nurture

Nurture is possibly the most complex and challenging of the three determinants. It deals with less understood areas such as the impact of lifestyle, culture and environment on human health implying changes in human behaviour. All national health delivery systems strive to persuade patients to be more physically active and more responsible for their own health. Yet they struggle to provide them with "response-ability" for their conditions: appropriate tools and services for meaningful, personalised and continuous information for patients/citizens to support disease management and healthier living are missing.

This calls for new large scale efforts to provide the basis for comprehensive knowledge management: deriving value (knowledge) from the existing, scattered scientific information around the EU. Fast development of tools and services to make this knowledge accessible and trusted will be essential. We need to innovate to empower each patient with this knowledge and hopefully affect his or her lifestyle, behaviour and interaction with the health delivery system.

In other words: we should provide patients with a *health compass* (or GPS *for Health*) with which they can successfully navigate their *health journeys*. Today, these look more like journeys in the dark or like travelling in the middle ages before transport infrastructure such as maps, signs and GPS were in place. For example, eHealth should enable patients and their carers to check who of their own health professionals can be reached first (online, by phone or at work) in order to avoid unnecessary travelling to emergency centres or optimise a needed intervention.

To conclude, it is important to point out that all three health determinants are interdependent. Progress in one feeds back to the others. Guidelines for healthy living or progress in understanding the impact of genomics cannot be made without proper evidence derived from daily patient care and associated health research. Similarly, progress in understanding our risks related to nature will impact on the lifestyle and on new generations of genomic medicine. The environment and lifestyle also impact on how our nature is expressed. To study the interplay of healthcare delivery, nature and nurture, and to exploit the full potential behind this holistic approach to human health, political institutions need to provide impetus and encourage this new avenue through support and implementation expenditures.

European Commission support of eHealth research and deployment

The ICT for Health unit of the European Commission DG Information Society and Media (DG INFSO) has been working on promoting ICT in healthcare for twenty years by investing in R&D projects (€650 Million)[8], publishing policy documents[9], supporting market validation (eTen Programme) and enabling large scale pilots such as epSOS (www.epsos.eu) through the Competitiveness and Innovation Programme (CIP). New tools for professionals have been developed and deployed in a variety of fields: medical imaging, minimally invasive diagnostics and surgery, information systems for storing and sharing data among healthcare organisations, personal health systems and telemedicine services that facilitate better management of patients with chronic diseases. The latest efforts in developing "lab on a chip" systems and artificial organs[10] will put new diagnostic power into the hands of general practitioners and bring increased quality of life to patients. The research and demonstration activities will continue in the future in close cooperation with Member States and other Commission services such as DG Health and Consumers (SANCO) and DG Regional Policy (REGIO).

Nature has been a focus of DG INFSO since 2001 when it began funding new forms of integrative research. The first initiative, called Biomedical Informatics[11] (http://bioinfomed.isciii.es/), combines developments in bio-, neuro- and medical informatics. In 2006, a new ambitious initiative, the *Virtual Physiological Human* (VPH) was launched. It aims to create multiscale patient-specific models and simulators of physiology and diseases (http://www.europhysiome.org). €200 Million in research support has been committed for the time span of 2006-2010, endowing the initiative with great potential. Bringing the advances of biology and genomics to the patient's bedside constitutes a huge challenge and calls for highly multidisciplinary approaches and global cooperation. DG INFSO cooperates in multiple projects with the US, Japan and New Zealand and works together closely with relevant genomics and system biology programmes of DG Research (RTD)[12].

So far, efforts in the field of nurture have been sporadic. DG INFSO has supported some research on ICT for disease prevention, understanding of risk factors, and on personal health systems for lifestyle management. However, studies on topics like environmental hazards are complex and are mostly carried out by public health research, with limitations in scope and time. New activities in this yet unexplored area of ICT for nurture need to be developed. At present, DG INFSO is actively seeking ideas in the community of researchers, policy makers, health professionals and, of course, patients and their representative organizations.

Tackling the full picture in an integrative, concise and comprehensive manner as outlined above requires a highly interdisciplinary approach and poses new challenges. The research areas involved each deal with their own concepts, methods, scientific language, knowledge representations, and journals. Research across disciplines is not sufficiently recognised and rewarded. Similarly, current medicine is mostly restricted to disease-focused interventions and fragmented into isolated specialties. It is based predominantly on aggregate evidence and not on target-specific knowledge of an individual in all diversity of his/her genomic profile, social context and environmental impacts. The European Commission recognises this challenge and supports research and infrastructure for interdisciplinary research in the seventh Framework Progamme (FP7).

The case of ICT for personalised care

The potential benefits of a holistic, interdisciplinary approach to health integrating the three determinants (healthcare, nature and nurture) can be exemplified through the case of ICT for personalised care enabling a new model of citizen-centred and wellness-focused health service delivery. In order to manage diseases, in particular chronic diseases, more efficiently and with better outcomes, it is necessary to provide continuity of care in terms of time and space and tools for proactive maintenance of health in the hands of empowered citizens/patients.

Continuous monitoring of vital health signs like heart rate, ECG, respiratory rate, blood oxygen levels etc., during the patients' daily activities and at their ordinary living and working environments can best substitute for costly frequent medical encounters. More comprehensive information becomes available to medical professionals assisting them to make accurate decisions and to offer increasingly effective care to their patients.

At the same time, this can only be achieved with the active involvement and participation of the patients in the management of their own health conditions. ICT can make this happen by providing monitoring devices to be used by the patients in their homes and services that promote regular patient-doctor interaction, adapted to the personal circumstances of the user, and available anywhere, anytime.

In order to cure a disease, we need to better understand not only the organ or area of the body in which the disease manifests itself, but also the human body as a whole. This idea is being slowly recognised and promoted in biomedical research, because the traditional reductionist approach has clear limits. It deals with each biological scale—at the organ, tissue, cell or protein level—and the respective functions as distinct from each other.

For example, to investigate human genetics, technologies have been developed which decode the entire genome of a human being into a numerical model, a sequence of numbers stored into a computer. This was the only way to cope with the complexity involved. Such a model alone cannot be extrapolated to comprehend a disease or whole organ functions. We must create the technology to code all structures and functions (*Physiome*[13]) of a human body into a coherent set of multiscale computer models. Such models of the human body are the only way to unravel the systemic complexity of disease-related processes. With the *Virtual Physiological Human* (VPH) initiative, Europe has taken the global lead in development and validation of multiscale models.

Ultimately, the knowledge acquired in chronic disease management, combined with secure re-use of electronic patient data for research and public health, will enable new services for continuous, personalised disease prevention. The provision of trusted (certified) individualised health information in an effective way will greatly improve health education, compliance to treatment, communication with treating physicians and lifestyle choices of each individual.

ICT-enabled personalised care comprises several target domains for research:

♦ **Efficient, personalised management of chronic diseases:** Many diseases affecting a growing proportion of the population are attributed to failing or compromised functions of vital organs such as the liver, pancreas, kidney, heart and lung. Patients rely on donor organs or mechanical systems to increase their chances of survival, albeit causing severe limitations in their mobility and way of life. Wearable or implantable artificial organs, representing the "real" convergence of ICT bio- and nanotechnologies, will support these patients in the long term, eliminating the need for donor transplants. Multilevel modelling and simulation tools will provide insights into the functionality of natural organs, even very complex ones like the liver. They will allow for the autonomous, personalised operation of an artificial organ adaptable to the individual's changing health and lifestyle circumstances. Advances in materials, biology and tissue engineering will help perform, in an artificial organ, vital functions at the cellular level like synthesis and detoxification. Micro- and nano-technologies will allow the implementation of such solutions into unobtrusive devices that both monitor the patient's health and offer the functionality of a natural organ.

♦ **Patient-centric services:** Family doctors are supposed to merge all information on a patient's health produced by specialists, and to monitor the general health of each of their patients. In principle, this would involve integrating clinical information with life style, environmental, demographic, and other personal information. In practice, this is done only to a limited extent, simply because there is no good way to organise this huge amount of information, extract a general understanding from it, and provide it to the patient and the General Practitioner. All of this needs to be done in such a way that patient-doctor communication, disease prevention and efficient use of healthcare resources are all optimised. The VPH initiative can provide such an organised scaffold, where the virtual model of the patient is regularly updated with relevant personal and clinical information, and reports about the patient's health are produced for the patient and the doctor. We could imagine an electronic health record where the folder is not only a pile of raw information, but a virtual model of the patient updated as the need arises and from which decision support and recommendations are generated.

♦ **Personalised, curative healthcare:** In order to accurately predict the patient's health risks and design tailored preventive interventions or acute therapies, the specific genetic predispositions, individual conditions, and environmental factors must be taken into account. Currently, this is very difficult, in fact impossible in most cases, but emerging technologies promise to bring this within reach for every General Practitioner. The pharmaceutical industry has already recognised that the future of the market is in personalised care and drugs. It is looking for ICT-based tools that can help better categorise patients and diseases based on conditions documented in electronic health records, biosignals from wearable systems, and VPH solutions providing better understanding of disease processes.

♦ **Preventive and predictive healthcare:** Many aspects of human physiology and pathology involving complex systemic interrelationships can presently be explained only in observational and statistical terms, whereas the cause and effect mechanisms mostly remain unknown. Predicting the impact of an action with the help of personalised models could drastically improve the accuracy and efficiency of diagnosis, treatment and monitoring, reduce complications and side effects, and minimise care to the necessary level. The new industry of simulators and services for predictive care has a huge potential not only within the healthcare institutions and research organisations but also as a tool adapted for individuals to manage their lifestyle.

♦ **New drugs and medical devices:** Today, drugs and devices are designed on a very limited base of knowledge and understanding of physiological processes. This necessitates extensive animal and clinical tests. While these will remain unavoidable, the VPH initiative promises to significantly improve the design process and thus reduce the extent and increase safety of animal and clinical experimentation. The EU has a traditional lead in the pharmaceutical and medical device market—such a competitive advantage will assure that the industry remains in Europe and benefits the EU economy.

To be successful, data generated in these different contexts, from telemonitoring to outcomes and results from simulation models need to be integrated and interconnected with (hospital, GPs, etc.) information systems and public health systems, or with new models developed in the nurture field. All of this must be based on advanced technology engineering and a solid, secure health information infrastructure.

The eHealth market—more than a new kid on the block

The synergy of the Health and ICT sectors brings great value not only to individual patients and health delivery systems, but also to the economy at large. eHealth has an acknowledged strong market potential due to growing demand in the face of changing demographics and disease patterns, and the challenged sustainability of health delivery systems. eHealth is recognised as the fastest growing pillar of the healthcare industries. It is currently estimated to be worth €60 billion, of which the EU market represents approximately one third[14]. eHealth can revive and boost innovation in traditional European health markets, in particular pharmaceutical products (valued at €206.5 billion based on retail prices[15]) and medical devices (for which annual European sales are estimated at €64 billion[16]), and is thus rightly acknowledged as the third pillar of the healthcare market.

To accelerate development of the market, eHealth was chosen as one out of six market sectors to be particularly supported by the European Commission's 'Lead Market Initiative' (LMI)[17]. A three-year eHealth action plan is currently underway, aiming to: Reduce market fragmentation and lack of interoperability through pilots, benchmarking, standardisation and certification; Improve legal certainty and consumer acceptance by disseminating information, best practice, guidelines, and implementing screening tools; and facilitate access to funding through increased visibility and training workshops, improved cooperation, pilots and guidance on financing.

If we do not address now the current high level of fragmentation and the challenges posed by the strong local customisation, the eHealth market is in danger of becoming a market failure. We must take proactive steps to turn it into a veritable *lead market* that will stimulate our economy.

Conclusion

In the future, breakthroughs in life and social sciences, genomics, proteomics, nano-biotechnology, biomedical informatics, and systems engineering will allow for highly focused person-specific, predictive and preventive diagnosis and therapy. ICT plays a crucial role in the advances of individual disciplines, but more importantly, it is the enabling mechanism for the synthesis and management of knowledge derived from research in all these domains so that it can be translated and applied to each one of us. Against this background, eHealth research should encompass all major factors impacting on human health and well-being beyond healthcare—not only the health delivery systems, but also the endogenous and exogenous health determinants, nature and nurture. Any research in the eHealth domain should focus on target-specific knowledge concerning an individual in all his/her diversity with respect to genomic profile, social context and environmental impacts.

In the face of urgent societal challenges in healthcare, the critical economic situation and the Lisbon agenda, a strong political engagement has developed seeking an increase of innovation capability in Europe. The European Commission and the European Union Member States are prepared to consider a *Large Scale Action* that ties closely together the separate lines of eHealth research, fosters innovation and provides support for large scale deployment[18].

There is a potential for a strong European leadership in pursuing an EU-wide large scale action on *technology and policy engineering in eHealth. This will* bring together health organisations and their information systems into a pan-European, coherent and secure health information infrastructure that supports patient care, public health, research and health reforms. Left alone, a continuous organic growth of eHealth systems such as hospital information systems and electronic health record systems will further fragment the eHealth market, leading to expensive, poor quality and unsafe products and services. In the same way as we have not left post office services or transport services to the mercy of "organic growth" we should support EU-wide agreements for core shared elements (interoperability) as the backbone of the future European health information area.

ILIAS IAKOVIDIS, PH.D., serves as Deputy Head of the ICT for Health unit of the European Commission, DG Information Society and Media. He is responsible for direction and scope of the European Union's eHealth research and innovation programs (~100 Mil Euro/year). He is coordinating the international cooperation in eHealth, in particular with U.S. Ilias is also working on EU policy and support to large-scale deployment with Member States as described in the eHealth Action Plan (COM 2004 356) of which he was the main co-author. Beyond the office duties, he continues to publish articles and books, teach graduate courses on medical informatics in EU and U.S., and give keynote lectures at major international conferences. In 2001 he was elected fellow of American College of Medical Informatics for his contribution to the field.

ENDNOTES

1. The views presented are those of the author and do not necessarily represent the official view of the European Commission on the subject.

2. Economic impact of interoperable electronic health records and ePrescription in Europe—EHR IMPACT, Study for the European Commission, http://www.ehr-impact.eu/cases/cases.html

3. Ibid, Regional EHR system Diraya in Andalusia, Spain—in progress

4. Iakovidis, I. (1998) Towards Personal Health Record: Current situation, obstacles and trends in implementation of Electronic Healthcare Records in Europe, In *International Journal of Medical Informatics,* vol. 52, no 123, pp 105 –117

5. SA Schroeder: We Can Do Better—Improving the Health of the American People. N Engl J Med 2007; 357:1221-8.

6. Benchmarking ICT use among General Practitioners in Europe, http://ec.europa.eu/information_society/eeurope/i2010/benchmarking/index_en.htm#eHealth_Benchmarking_(Phase_II) http://ec.europa.eu/information_society/eeurope/i2010/benchmarking/index_en.htm#NEW_Pilot_on_eHealth_indicators:_Benchmarking_ICT_use_among_General_Practitioners_in_Europe

7. See for instance Medcom figures at: www.medcom.dk/wm110197. A Medcom service, the Danish Health Data Network linking health and social care, was evaluated in 2006 with an estimated cumulative benefit by 2008 approximately € 1.4 billion, see eHealth is Worth it —The economic benefits of implemented eHealth solutions at ten European sites. Luxembourg: Office for Official Publications of the European Communities, 2006, http://europa.eu.int/information_society/activities/health/docs/publications/ehealthimpactsept2006.pdf

8. Iakovidis, I., Purcarea O. (2008) eHealth in Europe: from Vision to Reality. Studies in health technology and informatics 2008;134():163-8.

9. COM/2004/0356 final—e-Health - making healthcare better for European citizens: an action plan for a European e-Health Area {SEC(2004)539}: http://eur-lex.europa.eu/LexUriServ/LexUriServ.do?uri=CELEX:52004DC0356:EN:NOT

Commission Recommendation of 2 July 2008 on cross-border interoperability of electronic health record systems (notified under document number C(2008) 3282): http://eur-lex.europa.eu/LexUriServ/LexUriServ. do?uri=CELEX:32008H0594:EN:NOT

COM/2008/0689 final—Communication on telemedicine for the benefit of patients, healthcare systems and society: http://eur-lex.europa.eu/ LexUriServ/LexUriServ.do?uri=CELEX:52008DC0689:EN:NOT

10. Gatzoulis, L.; Iakovidis, I. (2007) Wearable and portable eHealth systems. Technological issues and opportunities for personalized care. IEEE engineering in medicine and biology magazine: the quarterly magazine of the Engineering in Medicine & Biology Society 2007;26(5):51-6

11. Maojo V., Iakovidis I., Martin-Sanchez F., Crespo J., Kulikowski C , Medical Informatics and Bioinformatics: European Efforts to facilitate synergy. J Biomed Inform. 2002.

12. Iakovidis, I., Le Dour, O., Karp, P. (2007) Biomedical Engineering and eHealth in Europe - Outcomes and Challenges of Past and Current EU Research Programs. Engineering in Medicine and Biology Magazine, IEEE, Volume 26, Issue 3, May-June 2007 Page(s):26 - 28

13. The physiome describes the physiological dynamics of the normal intact organism and is built upon information and structure (genome, proteome, and morphome). In its broadest sense, the physiome should define relationships from genome to organism and from functional behaviour to gene regulation.

14. eHealth Industry Stakeholders Group, reporting to i2010 Sub-Group on eHealth, 2008

15. EFPIA, The Pharmaceutical Industry in Figures, Key Data, 2009 Update, www.efpia.eu/Content/Default.asp?PageID=559&DocID=4883 (see p. 5)

16. Eucomed Medical Technology Brief, Key facts and Figures on the European Medical Technology Industry, 2007, www.eucomed.be/press/~/ media/pdf/tl/2008/portal/aboutindustry/medtechbrief2007.ashx

17. COM(2007)860 (21.12.2007). The specific eHealth Task Force report related to the LMI Communication can be accessed at: http://ec.europa. eu/information_society/activities/health/docs/publications/lmi-report-final-2007dec.pdf

18. COM(2009)116 of 13 March 2009 "A Strategy for ICT R&D and Innovation in Europe: Raising the Game," http://eur-lex.europa.eu/LexUriServ/ LexUriServ.do?uri=COM:2009:0116:FIN:EN:PDF

Chapter 7

Introducing Legal Aspect of the eHealth in Europe

Evika Karamagioli

Introduction

Although the health sector is a prime growth sector of European economies, growing faster and creating more new jobs than almost any other sector, financing healthcare is a key cost factor for European social security systems.

In parallel citizens' demand for best quality healthcare is increasing seriously. The same applies to the costs of managing chronic diseases, and the need for prolonged medical care for the ageing society. ICT-enabled solutions to health and healthcare, ranging from electronic prescriptions to electronic patient summaries or electronic health cards, which have being recognized as a key factor to better cope with these challenges improving the efficiency and effectiveness of health care. Simply, ICT represent an answer in order to guarantee quality standards in health for all. eHealth's innovative nature lies on the fact that it can connect different health professionals, regardless of their place of residence or their age.

However, in order for those kind of applications to benefit all citizens in the whole range of functions that affect the health sector—from the doctor to the hospital manager, via nurses, data processing specialists, social security administrators and of course the patients—coherent national plans and policies are required.

The European Union strongly supports these developments by adopting comprehensive action plans and funding technology-focused research in the eHealth field for more than 15 years. The co-financing allocated since the early 1990s and has reached €500 million, with a total budget about twice that amount. By 2010 it is expected to account for 5% of the total health budget of the European Union's Member States. It is clear therefore that the problem is not the lack of resources; it's the lack of coordination of how existing resources are actually used. By increasing out exchange of knowledge and experiences across Europe and globally, increased cost-effectiveness for the national investments are self-evident. The main strategic goal is to create political awareness and commitment at the highest levels; and to change the way eHealth is described, so that the added value for healthcare when implementing eHealth solutions is understandable and self-explaining for everyone outside the eHealth Community.

Many research results have now been tested and put into practice. These kinds of developments have contributed to the emergence of a new eHealth industry that has the potential to be the third largest industry in the health sector.

eHealth describes the application of ICTs across the whole range of functions that affect the health sector. eHealth tools or solutions include products, systems and services that go beyond simply Internet-based applications. They include tools for health authorities and professionals, as well as personalised health systems for patients and citizens. Examples include health information networks, electronic health records, telemedicine services, personal wearable and portable communicable systems, health portals, as well as many other information and communication technology-based tools assisting prevention, diagnosis, treatment, health monitoring, and lifestyle management.

When combined with organizational changes and the development of new skills, eHealth can help to deliver better care for less money within citizen-centred health delivery systems. It thus plays a clear role in the European Union's "eEurope Strategy," and it's key to achieve stronger growth and create highly qualified jobs in a dynamic, knowledge-based economy—a vision that was set out by the Lisbon European Council on March 2000.

It is apparent that eHealth is not just about technology, but about changing the everyday practice of healthcare for every healthcare professional and every patient. Unfortunately the legal and regulatory environment of eHealth has not progressed as rapidly as technology; and the emerged key issue in the European level now is whether and to what extent the legal and regulatory environment of eHealth interferes with public health policy and whether it should be regulated separately from the more "traditional" healthcare. Thus, there is a necessity in leaving the period of technological development and enter the next phase, which should be focused on organizational change. The work of improving information flows and continuity of care with the help of ICT support systems will not be able to reach its full potential until working methods, processes and the culture in healthcare are adapted to this new environement—and adapted to meet the individual needs of the patients.

This chapter will examine whether the existing European legislation is sufficient to cover the use of eHealth tools in the provision of healthcare to citizens; if and how EU legislation on data protection, *product and services liability, and trade and competition law* applies along with physician-patient (healthcare provider-citizen) relationships on the Internet. Lastly it will highlight specific trends on eHealth from several countries.

An overview of the EU strategy

In 2004, the Commission adopted the eHealth action plan—which covers everything from electronic prescriptions and health cards to new information systems that reduce waiting times and errors—to facilitate a more harmonious and complementary European approach to eHealth.

As EU Commissioner on Health, A. Vassiliou stated, "The purpose is not to question the MS's competence in determining how eHealth should be applied at their level. However, their efforts should be coordinated." Thus, the plan sets out the steps needed for widespread adoption of eHealth technologies across the EU by 2010 and calls on Member States to develop tailored national and regional eHealth strategies to respond to their own specific needs. In the framework of both the Lisbon strategy and the i2010 initiative, eHealth is a way of accelerating the achievement of a knowledge-based economy. Cultural differences, varying population profiles and geography all mean that regional and national health policies have to be developed individually. Where the EU becomes involved, under the action plan, it is to encourage each health authority to learn from the experiences of others. Through sharing ideas and experiences across Europe, all European citizens can benefit more rapidly from efficient and reliable eHealth systems.

The action plan sets out a series of targets to be met in the years up to 2010. New technological applications often need new methods of assessment before Member States' authorities can give the green light to their introduction into health service use. On the basis of best practices identified across Europe, all Member States should adopt procedures for testing and accreditation of eHealth tools and services by the end of 2007. Faster rollout of high-speed internet access, on which so many of the tools are based, is a crucial development if we are to fully exploit the widespread benefits of eHealth.

Simultaneously, the Union states that promoting the accessibility of eHealth services, particularly to groups which are least likely to have easy internet access, such as the elderly, disabled or unemployed, who are often those who have most need of health services, is a top priority of the action plan.

eHealth is also an integral component of the EU's i2010 policy framework which seeks to promote an open and competitive digital economy, ICT-related research, as well as applications to improve social inclusion, public services and quality of life.

Given that Public Health is limited by the principle of subsidiarity[1] it is clear that EU Member States have the prime responsibility to protect and improve the health of their citizens. As part of that responsibility, it is for them to decide on the organisation and delivery of health services and medical care. However, when exercising these competences, Member States nonetheless have to comply with Community law. An example of such collaboration on this area is the creation of several projects which have been launched during 2008, namely the epSOS Large Scale Pilot and the CALLIOPE Thematic Network. By these projects, the ambition to move from strategies of eHealth to services are finally being fullfilied.

There are however a number of examples in the health area on which Member States cannot act alone effectively and where cooperative action at the EU level is indispensable, especially regarding issues with a cross-border dimension or relating to the free movement of persons within the internal EU market. Both existing and emerging incompatibilities between Member State's legislation and European case-law concerning healthcare undermine the development of cross-border services and produce distortions of competition.

Several legal issues were particularly raised in the aforementioned *2004 Action Plan for a European eHealth Area* which proposes that by 2009 the European Commission shall provide a framework for greater legal certainty of eHealth products and services liability within the context of existing product liability legislation.

According to the plan there is a need to set a baseline for a standardised European qualification for e-Health services, both in clinical and administrative settings. Furthermore, there is a need to define with more certainty the liability of eHealth products and eHealth services, within the context of existing *product liability legislation*. ICT developments should contribute to a safer working environment for practitioners; and greater legal certainty with regard to eHealth services within the context of freedom of movement of people, goods and services is increasingly necessary.

By the end of 2009, the European Commission, in collaboration with the Member States, should undertake activities to:

♦ Set a baseline for a standardised European qualification for e-Health services in clinical and administrative settings.

♦ Provide a framework for greater legal certainty of eHealth products and services liability within the context of existing *product liability legislation*.

♦ Improve information for patients, health insurance schemes and providers regarding the rules applying to the assumption of the costs of eHealth services.

♦ Promote eHealth with a view to reduce occupational accidents and ill-nesses as well as support preventive actions in the face of the emergence of new workplace risks.

Thus the top priority is to restart, at the EU level, the revision process of existing regulatory framework by systematic screening and impact assessment. To this purpose, the Commission services are carefully examining the possibility whether additional regulatory provisions are necessary or whether current provisions are sufficient to ensure legal and regulatory certainty.

Legal issues to consider

Solving legal issues is a key element in any eHealth system development. Personal medical and clinical data are for most citizens very sensitive information and ought to be accessible only by trustworthy health or care staff. Thus, especially when planning large-scale data exchange networks with numerous health and social care actors, such as the EU's eHealth system, it is essential to ensure absolute data privacy and security.

Legislation already implemented or under discussion in Member States on these matters, helps in developing appropriate technical features and provides clarity about organisational procedures. New technologies open up new opportunities but also new risks. In order to protect citizens, regardless of whether they act as patients or health professionals, the legislation that is existent in most countries may have to be reviewed and adapted to the new opportunities—and threats—created by eHealth solutions.

Data Protection, Privacy, Confidentiality

eHealth applications, whatever their nature, frequently involve the processing of information related to an identified or identifiable "subject," the patient. Such information legally is known as personal data and is subject to the *data protection legislation* of the European Union. In Europe, such data are protected by legal rules found in a number of legal sources. More specifically, the fundamental right to the protection of personal data is based on *Article 8* of the *European Convention for the Protection of Human Rights and Fundamental Freedoms* and on *Article 8* of the *EU Charter of Fundamental Rights* as well as the *Directive on Data Protection* (Dir. 95/46/EC), which now has been adopted into national data protection legislation across the EU. This Directive, however, has also another purpose: To allow the free movement of personal data within the European Union in the context of the internal market.

The basic principle behind this Directive in this content, is that if a piece of information can be linked to a person either by reasonable simple means, by or with the help of a third person, then the data is considered as identifiable and, therefore, fall into the range of the aforementioned Directive. For example the laboratory results of a blood sample test, will be covered by this legislation if the identification of the originator of the blood is possible using reasonable means.

The data protection rules fall primarily into the responsibility and jurisdiction of the data controller—the person who decides the purpose and the means of the data processing and who has the legal duty to ensure that data are handled appropriately. In most professional cases, this will be a senior staff member who is named as the person responsible for data collection and storage by an organization. In the case of small companies or self-employed individuals (such as many General Practitioners), the data controller generally will be the person who has legal and tax liability for the organization.

However data concerning a person's health, religion, trade union activity, as well as data revealing racial or ethnic origin and judicial information, are amongst the data defined by the Directive as especially *sensitive* and, therefore, are subject to special rules. These data are capable by their nature of infringing fundamental freedoms or privacy of the data subject (patient) and, therefore, should not be processed.

This is not an absolute rule in any of the EU countries as they all accept, by principle, that medical data may be collected or processed only for certain purposes and following certain guidelines such as: a) After the citizen's/patient's (data subject) explicit and informed consent, b) In the case of physical or mental incapability of the data subject in consenting for his/her data processing, there is a need to protect his/her vital interest, c) In the case of any health professional or any other subject with equivalent position which controls or processes medical data, he/she is obliged of professional secrecy concerning these data for the purposes of preventive medicine, medical diagnosis, the provision of care or treatment, or the management of healthcare services.

Patient Rights

Concerning patient rights and eHealth the EC due to the low take-up of telemedicine applications in real-life medicine tried to identify the barriers and trigger factors for greater use of eHealth applications and issued Communications towards those ends; such as the Communication on Telemedicine for the Benefit of Patients. According to this Communication MS should have assessed and adapted their national regulations by the end of 2011 enabling wider access to telemedicine services. Issues such as accreditation, liability, reimbursement and privacy should be addressed.

Additionally, EC in its recent proposal for a Directive on the application of patients' rights in cross-border healthcare, referred also to eHealth. Article 16 of this proposal stipulates that the Commission shall adopt specific measures necessary for achieving the interoperability of information and communication technology systems in the healthcare field, applicable whenever MSs decide to introduce them (Callens, 2009).

Product and Service Liability and Consumer Protection

It is clear that the provision of eHealth products, systems, and services must comply with certain levels of quality. There are various rules that provide guarantees for any damages caused from sub-standard products or services, in favour of the consumer. Those do not apply exclusively to eHealth, but instead are applied to a general context of service provision and product delivery, whether by traditional or via electronic means. The concept of the eHealth product is sometimes difficult to understand because, in practice, most eHealth products either will be software packages and interfaces (electronic health record, decision support tool) or they might be hardware devices with embedded software (radio frequency identification location trackers for locating people and objects; remotely controlled medical devices). Hence there is a broad definition of what "consists" an eHealth product or service, so as to include anything that is sold to a medical practitioner or directly to a consumer (patient) that uses an Internet for his/hers purchases. According to this, an eHealth product might be a medical electronic record to be used by a doctor, or a monitoring device that includes a web-based interface, or even just a simple health information portal.

In order for the EC (European Commission) to reassure product liability, there are specific measures that have been applied in the form of Directives. *The General Product Safety Directive* establishes a general safety requirement for any product put on the market for consumers; including eHealth products. The national legislation based on EC's *General Product Liability Directives* ensures that the purchaser has the right to be compensated if the consumer goods are not fit for the purpose sold; the same concept exists also to national legislation based on Directive on the *Sale of Consumer Goods*. According to the above, when eHealth products are sold as consumer goods, the provider must deliver goods as described in the contract of sale.

Any eHealth device placed on the market, which is designated by its manufacturer as a medical device, will be subject to the specific additional rules regarding medical devices. The medical devices sector is covered by three directives, covering a wide scope of products. The first Directive, (90/385/EC), deals with active implantable medical devices (ex. pace-makers etc.), the second Directive, (93/42/EC), deals with medical devices in general, while the third Directive, (98/79/EC), deals with in vitro diagnostic medical devices.

National, international, and European bodies are developing standards that apply to eHealth products. Examples include the *European Committee for Standardization* (CEN), standard for Electronic Health Records (EHRs), the

American *Health Level Seven* (HL7) standard for EHR, or the industry standard for the Digital Imaging and Communications in Medicine (DICOM). While these standards are not legally binding, they do provide a baseline against which disputes about the quality of an eHealth product, covered by a standard, might be assessed.

Directive 85/374/EC on *Defective Products* will apply to eHealth products in the same way as it applies to any other product sold on the European market. This Directive aims to ensure a high level of consumer protection against damage caused to health or property by a defective product. It also aims to reduce the disparities between national liability laws, which distort competition and restrict the free movement of goods.

On another end, the Directive (2005/36/EC) on the recognition of professional qualifications, guarantees that persons having acquired in a MS will have access to the same profession and be able to pursue it in another member state with the same rights as nationals, unless the latter MS has laid down any non-discriminatory conditions of pursuit, provided that these are objectively justified and proportionate.

There is currently no general European harmonisation of liability rules for services in which no defect can be found in a device. Therefore, liability for services is governed by ordinary rules of law applicable in the Member States. An exception to this may exist if a service is supplied wholly by electronic means, in which case the eCommerce Directive (2000/31/EC) might apply. Therefore, any eHealth services provide via the Internet will be subject to the national legislation derived from the eCommerce Directive of the EU, with the precondition that they meet the qualities of an information society service.

An information society service entails any service that is normally provided for remuneration, at a distance, by electronic means, and at the individual request of a recipient of services (such as through the Internet). It covers services between enterprises or between enterprises and consumers, which are paid directly from the recipient (online transactions) or those financed by indirect means, such as advertising income or sponsoring such as:

- ◆ Websites of doctors promoting their activities;
- ◆ Online selling of medicines (ePharmacy);
- ◆ Online advice that does not require the physical examination of the patient if a fee is paid or if it is financed by advertising or sponsorship;
- ◆ Online databases of information accessible for medical professionals or consumers if a fee is paid or if it is financed by advertising or sponsorship (even indirectly).

This principle of transparency of the site provider is included within the Commission's *Communication on Quality Criteria for Health-related Websites* (COM 2002/667). These criteria seek to increase the reliability of health-related websites and also include other quality criteria that health-related websites should comply with, such as transparency of the purpose of the website, respect of privacy, accessibility adapted to the target audience, etc. Those quality criteria may serve as reference in the development of quality initiatives for health-related websites.

Aspects of Trade and Competition Law

Both existing and emerging disparities in Member States' legislation and case-law concerning healthcare, prevent the smooth functioning of the internal market, in particular by impairing the development of cross-border services and producing distortions of competition.

Since health services are, in most EU countries, funded through some form of taxation, and organised to some degree by public bodies, the extent to which competition law applies to them is somewhat unclear and may be limited. More explicitly, it is unclear in how far the rules of competition apply at all to publicly funded bodies, how far the concept of Services of General Interest apply to health services, and the extent to which health services are, on the basis of the rules on *Services of General Economic Interest* as provided for in the Treaty, exempted from the provisions of European competition law.

Historically and socially, the provision of healthcare services has been hidden from the area of competition law not only because of its public nature, but also because healthcare generally is conceived as an intellectual service provided by professionals whose services comprise a range of skills not classified into separate activities subject to competition. As a result, healthcare, historically, has not attracted the attention of competition lawyers to any significant extent. However, this should not cause any problems since an eHealth company is not necessarily any different from a hotel group or a car manufacturer. Yet, the context in which eHealth organisations operate might make them considerably different from other organisations, not least because an eHealth company will, in many cases, be selling its services not directly to the consumer, but to a public health services provider who, in turn, makes eHealth services available to patients and citizens in the course of their usual provision of care.

For the health sector, it is important to think not only about the application of the rules on abuse of dominant position, and the possible exemptions of Services of General Economic Interest (SGEIs), but also about state aid, since many health service providers will be funded directly through state aid. Most healthcare providers are unlikely to be legally classified as undertakers of an economic activity, since they are supplying goods and services in the execution of an exclusively social function; meaning that this function is built on a non-profit making basis, on the principle of solidarity and where the entitlement to services is not dependent on the amount of contributions. Their interactions with private bodies from which goods or services are purchased for the purposes of providing healthcare will not be subject to the rules on abuse of dominant position. A healthcare provider, however, operating outside those strict criteria, could well be classified as an undertaker of economic activities and, therefore, subject to competition law.

Article 87 states that any aid granted by a Member State, or is funded by state resources, in any form whatsoever, can be considered incompatible with the rules of the common market, in the case that it distorts or threatens to distort competition by favouring certain undertakings or the production of certain goods.

Despite the absolute character of Article 87, the European Commission has the power to decide where state aid has a social character and is granted to individual consumers (e.g., state aid to assist consumers who have suffered loss due to the collapse of a major industry) or where state aid is used to repair the damages caused by natural disasters. In the second case, such state aid may be considered as compatible with the common market. The Commission also may permit some specific aids.

In general, any project of state aid must be notified in advance to the Commission. Some state aid, however, in the form of public service compensation that is granted to certain undertakings, and entrusted with the operation of Services of General Economic Interest (e.g., hospitals), are not considered as incompatible with the common market and need not to be notified.

Patient mobility and cross-border medical reimbursement

Despite the significant progress achieved in the use of ICT in health area, the reimbursement for cross-border services in eHealth is not regulated at the EU level. The mechanism used for cross-border care reimbursement in the EU is based on Regulations, on coordination of social security systems and on the Internal Market rules concerning the free provision of services, which have been clarified by the European Court of Justice. Although the existing regulations provide a well-established tool that has ensured social protection for workers, tourists and patients travelling within the EU, the system needs improvement in order to exploit the great potential for eHealth applications for the enhancement of safer, more efficient cross-border care in which, in many cases, neither patient nor practitioner would need to move his/her actual location. Every effort should, therefore, be made to ensure that the potential revision of legal provisions around patient mobility is fully aligned with the use of eHealth goods and services, to deliver healthcare across borders.

Indicative legislation from EU countries

In every EU country we can find general legislation or general regulations on data protection, confidentiality and telecommunications, digital signatures and device liability. Few of them have currently started to introduce specific legal acts on eHealth related matters, such as medical privacy and data ownership rights, ePrescribing, legal framework for health ICT standards or Health Telematics.

Here are some examples of general legislation/regulations on data protection from different EU Member States; France has one of the most advanced legal systems in the health sector. Legislation exists in the area of data protection, telemedicine, eHealth service provision and Health-IT product liability, as well as Electronic Health Record. Indicative measures comprise:

◆ The "Commission Nationale Informatique et Libertés" (CNIL) law of January 1978, following with the European Legislation which prohibits data processing without consent of the data subject, except for data absolutely necessary to the health professionals in charge of treating the person concerned, or those related to health service management and in which cases professional secrecy is required.

◆ The "Ordonnances Juppé" of April 1996, which organises the secured electronic infrastructure for the health system, based on authentication of the insured persons and the health professionals, as well as the usage of a secured network based on internet standards to exchange electronic information.

◆ The Medical Privacy Act (4 February 2002), which details the ownership rights of the patient to his or her data, whereby their transmission is authorised only between health professionals treating the same patient, and only with the patient's prior consent (article L1110-4).

◆ The legal framework for health ICT standards is the Healthcare Insurance Act of August 2004 (Loi n°2004/810 sur l'Assurance Maladie), in which Articles 32, 33, 34, 67 are related to telemedicine. This law also provides for the creation of the "Dossier Médical Personnel" (DMP, Personal Medical Record), on behalf of the patient, in order to facilitate the continuity of his/her healthcare. A dedicated structure, the GIP (Public Interest Group) DMP, was created in April 2005 to design, supervise and organize the deployment of the DMP. Furthermore, the "Dossier Pharmaceutique" (prescription dossier), was created by law in early 2007 in connection with the DMP.

Another example is Norway, which shows a worth-mentioning progress in this area. Legislative research initiated in spring 2006 to describe ways in which the *Norwegian Personal Data Act*, the *Health Registries Act* and other acts are hindering progress in eHealth. This may lead to proposals for new legislation. In August 2006 the Directorate launched a code of conduct, defining how the different health care organisations should treat patient and health information in order to comply with the national and European Data Protection Act.

Final example is Sweden, where an ongoing review of legislation on information management in the health care sector is conducted by the Patient Data Inquiry. In Sweden many of the national eHealth solutions are now in the final stages of development. The long awaited National Patient Summary is now being implemented in region by region, and a modern legal framework has been established since July 2008 by the new Patient Data Act (Hägglund 2009).

Potential Risks

Based on the article by Louis Marinos and Barbara Daskala, even if the benefits of eHealth are clear, there are, however, risks entailed that cannot be ignored. More explicitly, the EU Agency ENISA (European Network and Information Security Agency) has released a report presenting potential Emerging and Future Risks (EFR) in a possible remote health monitoring and treatment scenario, having deployed its recently developed framework on identifying risks of emerging and new applications and/or technologies (EFR Framework). eHealth is the first scenario that has been developed as they state in their article and analyzed by a group of interdisciplinary experts. The report identifies 14 potential risks and underlined the importance of a cautionary approach towards eHealth solutions. The assets, i.e what this framework aims to protect against these risks include first and foremost the human life, human rights and social values, autonomy, the national health care system, mobility of citizens and their personal data (Marinos & Daskala 2009).

Conclusion

eHealth is not just about technology but about changing the everyday practice of healthcare for every healthcare professional and every patient. When combined with organizational changes and the development of new skills, eHealth can help to deliver better care for less money within citizen-centred health delivery systems. It thus plays a clear role in the European Union's *eEurope strategy*, and is key to achieve stronger growth and create highly qualified jobs in a dynamic, knowledge-based economy—which comes in accordance with the vision set out by the Lisbon European Council on March 2000.

EU Member States have the prime responsibility for protecting and improving the health of their citizens. As part of that responsibility, it is for them to decide on the organisation and delivery of health services and medical care. However, when exercising these competences, Member States nonetheless have to comply with Community law and simultaneously this is the reason why, the EU with its Recommendations and Communications complements the initiatives adopted at the national level (Vassiliou 2009).

There are, however, a number of examples in the health area on which Member States cannot act alone effectively and where cooperative action at the EU level is indispensable, especially regarding issues with a cross-border dimension or relating to the free movement of persons within the internal EU market. Both existing and emerging disparities in Member States' legislation and case-law, concerning healthcare impair the development of cross-border services and produce distortions of competition.

Additionally, the legal and regulatory environment of eHealth has not progressed as rapidly as technology, and a key issue in the European sphere is whether and to what extent it interferes with public health national policy and should be regulated separately from the more "traditional" healthcare; as well as to what extend is national or European affair?

The processing of personal data for example may vary due to the different national specifications and the diverse transposition and implementation of the relevant European Directive. It is, therefore, important to consider whether the EU should adopt special interpretative guidelines to the provisions of Directive 95/46/EC, or other actions to promote proper implementation and improve enforcement of the Directive, so that eHealth-related stakeholders are made more aware of the rules on personal data processing in the field of eHealth.

Finally, issues concerning liability for the quality and safety of eHealth products are still rather new, and much uncertainty exists about who is liable for what and how liability is split among different service providers in the eHealth continuum; especially when this uncertainty relates to cross-border healthcare beyond that already provided by international private law. In this context, based on the Directive on liability for defective products, efficient protection for civil liability against defective goods and services must meet the objectives of spreading fairly the risks inherent in a modern high-technology society, protecting consumers' health, stimulating innovation, securing undistorted competition, and facilitating trade. Lastly, one can conclude that eHealth as a key part of the eEurope strategy and due to its cross-border dimension, constitutes an answer to the different socio-economic objectives set out by the EU. Therefore the Union as a whole and MSs separately "should continue to act together and promote expansion of eHealth, within the framework respecting health data confidentiality" (Vassiliou 2009).

Ms. Evika Karamagioli currently serves as Deputy Director at Gov2, an internationally recognized technology NGO, in the field of eDemocracy and eParticipation. Prior posts include Project Manager in the ICT for Policy and Citizen Engagement Unit of Gov2u from 2005-2008. Gov2U, Grants & Research Coordinator in the Greek NGO access2democracy, Scientific Associate at the Centre for European Constitutional Law Themistocles and Dimitris Tsatsos Foundation, and responsible for European Project Management at the Athens Bar Association, Greece. She has extensive experience in designing and managing research projects funded from International and National Development Agencies in the areas of e-democracy, eParticipation and eInclusion. She also contributed as a researcher in the elaboration of a series of studies concerning public administration modernization and eGovernment. From 2007-2008 she was involved as an independent expert in the Ad hoc committee on eDemocracy of the Council of Europe (CAHDE). She is currently a reviewer in the European Journal of ePractice. She holds a Masters in International Security and Defence from the University of Grenoble, France and a Masters in Crisis Management from Athens University, Greece. She is currently a Ph.D. candidate at the University Paris 8, France. She has published extensively on the subjects of eDemocracy and human rights and ICT.

ENDNOTES

1. The principle of subsidiarity is defined in Article 5 of the Treaty establishing the European Community. It is intended to ensure that decisions are taken as closely as possible to the citizen and that constant checks are made as to whether action at Community level is justified in the light of the possibilities available at national, regional or local level. Specifically, it is the principle whereby the Union does not take action (except in the areas which fall within its exclusive competence) unless it is more effective than action taken at national, regional or local level. It is closely bound up with the principles of proportionality and necessity, which require that any action by the Union should not go beyond what is necessary to achieve the objectives of the Treaty.

REFERENCES

Article 5 of the Treaty establishing the E.C. (subsidiarity principle)

Article 152 of the Treaty establishing the E.C. (Public Health)

European Parliament resolution of 23 May 2007 on the impact and consequences of the exclusion of health services from the Directive on services in the internal market (2006/2275(INI))

e-Health—making healthcare better for European citizens: an action plan for a European e-Health Area COM(2004) 356 final Available at: http://ec.europa.eu/information_society/doc/qualif/health/COM_2004_0356 _F_EN_ACTE.pdf

Ageing well in the Information Society—An i2010 Initiative Action Plan on Information and Communication Technologies and Ageing COM(2007) 332 final

eHealth Action Plan, Progress Report. Available at: http://ec.europa.eu/information_society/activities/health/docs/policy/ehealth-ap-prog-report2005.pdf

Database of European eHealth priorities and strategies (Empirica). Available at: http://www.ehealth-era.org/database/database.html

European Observatory on Health Systems and Policies, Health Systems in Transition (HiT) country profiles. Available at: http://www.euro.who.int/observatory/Hits/TopPage

European Observatory on Health Systems and Policies, Patient Mobility in the European Union. Learning from experience. Available at: http://www.euro.who.int/observatory/Publications/20060522_4

Pilot on eHealth indicators: 'Benchmarking ICT use among General Practitioners in Europe (Empirica), Final report. Available at: http://ec.europa.eu/information_society/eeurope/i2010/docs/benchmarking/gp_survey_final_report.pdf

Legally eHealth, Study on Legal and Regulatory Aspects of eHealth, Available at: http://www.ehma.org/projects/default.asp?NCID=140

Directive 95/46/EC of the European Parliament and of the Council of 24 October 1995 on the protection of individuals with regard to the processing of personal data and on the free movement of such data. Available at:

http://eurlex.europa.eu/LexUriServ/LexUriServdo?uri=CELEX:31995L0046:
EN:HT ML

eHealth ERA report 2007 eHealth priorities and strategies in European
countries. Available at http://www.ehealth-era.org/documents/
2007ehealth-era-countries.pdf'

Accelerating the Development of the eHealth Market in Europe', eHealth
Taskforce report 2007 Luxembourg: Office for Official Publications of the
European Communities, 2007 ISBN-978-92-79-07288-8 Available at:
http://www.ehealtheurope.net/img/case_studies0334/LMI-report.pdf

European Council (2006): Council Conclusions on Common values and
principles in European Union Health Systems. Document (2006/C 146/01),
published in the Official Journal of the European Union on 22 June 2006

European Commission: Information Society and Health: Linking European
Policies. Luxembourg: Office for Official Publications of the EC, 2006.

Wilson, P., Leitner, Ch. and Moussalli, A. (2004): Mapping the Potential
of eHealth, Empowering the citizen through eHealth tools and services.
Maastricht: European Institute of Public Administration.

Weerasinghe D. Electronic Healthcare: First International Conference, eHealth
2008, London, September 8-9, 2008, Revised Selected Papers (Lecture Notes
of the Institute ... and Telecommunications Engineering) (Paperback)

Vasisiliou, A., "eHealth, for a better quality of healthcare", European
Commission (EC), European Files, May 2009, N°17 "eHealth in Europe.
[Online] Available at: http://ec.europa.eu/information_society/newsroom/cf/
itemlongdetail.cfm?item_id=5012 or http://www.epractice.eu/files/The%20
European%20Files%20-%20eHealth%20in%20Europe%20-%20EN.pdf

Hägglund, G., "It's time to put eHealth on the political agenda!", European
Commission (EC), European Files, May 2009, N°17 "eHealth in Europe.
[Online] Available at: http://ec.europa.eu/information_society/newsroom/cf/
itemlongdetail.cfm?item_id=5012 or http://www.epractice.eu/files/The%20
European%20Files%20-%20eHealth%20in%20Europe%20-%20EN.pdf

Callens, S., "Legal Basis of eHeath and Telemedicine", European Commission
(EC), European Files, May 2009, N°17 "eHealth in Europe. [Online] Available
at: http://ec.europa.eu/information_society/newsroom/cf/itemlongdetail.
cfm?item_id=5012 or http://www.epractice.eu/files/The%20European%20
Files%20-%20eHealth%20in%20Europe%20-%20EN.pdf

Marinos, L., and Daskala, B., "e-Health: the benefits are clear, but the risks entailed cannot be ignored", European Commission (EC), European Files, May 2009, N°17 "eHealth in Europe. [Online] Available at: http://ec.europa. eu/information_society/newsroom/cf/itemlongdetail.cfm?item_id=5012 or http://www.epractice.eu/files/The%20European%20Files%20-%20eHealth %20in%20Europe%20-%20EN.pdf

Chapter 8

Introducing the eHealth Status of Greece

Korinna Zoi Karamagkioli, M.D.

Introduction

The benefits of eHealth for an impregnable and more efficient health sector have long been recognized by expert stakeholders. For individuals, eHealth brings new possibilities in terms of increasing quality and effectiveness of services. eHealth provides completely new methods for the treatment of chronic or rare diseases. In the European context, it can facilitate implementation of cross-border healthcare and contribute to continuity of care. For society, eHealth means a challenge for interoperability, e-literacy, and accessibility of new technologies. It is a great opportunity for research and development. For economy, eHealth offers solutions that can bring enormous savings. If properly deployed, eHealth can contribute to the transformation of the health sector, substantially change the business model of healthcare facilities, and impact the behaviour of health insurance institutions.

Greece has to be considered rather a laggard in terms of eHealth as it scores below the EU27 average with regard to most indicators included in the survey. This concerns both the availability of ICT infrastructure (computer, Internet) and the use of ICT for different eHealth-related purposes. In terms of infrastructure, 79% of the Greek GP practices use a computer. 66% of practices dispose of an Internet connection. In Greece, broadband connections have not yet arrived in force; they are, however, already used in 44% of GP practices. When it comes to the use of eHealth solutions, Greece shows results that are somewhat below the EU27 averages.

Greece displays its best eHealth performance in the area of patient data storage. Yet even here, usage rates lie below the EU27 average. Greece ranks fairly well with relation to the storage of medical patient data, which is used on average by more than two-thirds of GPs. In relation to the storage of radiological data, Greece even scores slightly above the EU27 average of 34%. The rather low usage rates of eHealth applications in Greece might be due to the only quite recent development of an encompassing health strategy.

The national eHealth roadmap that has been drafted in 2006 aims at the establishment of a National Health Information System including the introduction of Electronic Health Records. Pilot implementations and demonstrations are planned for the 2007–2012 period. The necessary networking infrastructure—including standards, a national health portal, health insurance smart cards, various electronic information systems, etc.—will, therefore, only become available on a wider scale in the upcoming years.

The overall objective of this chapter is to provide a comprehensive overview of eHealth sector in Greece.

The public health sector perspective

A recent study of the Observatory of the Greek Information Society reveals new facts regarding the utilization of Information and Communication Technologies (ICT) in the areas of Health and Welfare in Greece. The study mainly focuses on the availability and usage of computers and the Internet in the Greek Public Health Sector as well as on the digital literacy of medical practitioners, nurses and related staff. Particular emphasis has also been placed on the assessment of ICT-related Projects, which took place within the Third Community Support Framework (CSF).[1]

According to this study, the Greek Public Health Sector is characterized by a high ICT penetration level: the majority of health personnel (61%) has computer access at the place of employment. However, only 34% use computers to support their work, and only a few of them on a daily basis. Though 87% of the employees know how to use a computer, only 23% own a relevant certification. A total of 54% has access to the Internet, however, only 18% utilizes an email account issued by the respective authority.

Another key finding of the study constitutes the fact that the personnel is already aware of the importance of ICT in the Health Sector. Applications that are considered to be of critical importance include those related to electronic Patient Records (79%), eHealth Cards (75%) and Health Information Systems (74%). Furthermore, the necessity to introduce eProcurement Systems has been pointed out, mainly by IT personnel, yet not by top level management staff.

Regarding the contribution of ICT to the Public Health sector, the majority (80%) of IT and administration staff considers it as positive. The same also applies to 76% of the medical personnel. ICT is positively perceived by citizens as it contributes to avoid mistakes, ensure faster and improved service delivery as well as shorter complains processing times.

Practitioners' perspective

ICT infrastructure (computer, internet) entails:

- ◆ The availability of one or more computers in the practice;
- ◆ A connection in the Internet; and
- ◆ The availability of a broadband connection.

When it comes to the use of ehealth solutions, Greece shows results below the EU27 average. In terms of infrastructure, 79% of the Greek GP practices use a computer. 66% of practices dispose of an Internet connection. In Greece, broadband connections have not yet arrived in force; they are, however, already used in 44% of GP practices. Decision Support Systems are used by 12% of Greek GPs, which corresponds to one of the lowest usage rate with respect to this indicator in the EU27. Patient data transfer has as yet not very much arrived on the agenda of Greek GPs. The use of electronic networks for the transmission of medical patient data is not well established. Only 4% of the GP practice participating in the survey reported having exchanged medical data with other care providers via some sort of network.

Another very important aspect ePrescribing is still not a reality in most European member states. This holds true for Greece as well where only 2% of GPs having participated in the survey reported using ePrescribing.

An explanation for the rather low usage rates of eHealth applications in Greece might be due to the only quite recent development of an encompassing eHealth strategy. In Greece more than three-quarters (79%) of GP practices have a computer. Furthermore, most GP practices fulfill the infrastructural prerequisite for the implementation of eHealth applications. However, they are not properly equipped so as to make the best use of eHealth solutions. Prerequisites for health applications are a connection to the internet or any other dedicated network. In Greece 44% of the practices use a broadband connection, and it leads a small groups of countries were less than 50% of GP practices have such an access. In the matter of electronic patient data storage, Greece is one of the laggards. However, at least one type of individual medical patient data is stored.

The types of data stored most often include basic diagnoses (74%), medical history (73%) and medications (71%). Basic medical parameters, lab results, symptoms, examinations and results, vital signs measurements and treatment outcomes are all registered by more than 60% of GP practices. Radiological data storage is practiced by 42% as compared to the EU27 average of 34%. Neither in Europe as a whole, nor in Greece has the electronic exchange of patient data via the internet or other networks established. Telemonitoring is used only in

1% of the practices in Greece, but even in Sweden which has the highest usage, only 9% of GPs report the use of it. One out of five GPs use only coded data for the storage of electronic data, slightly below the EU27 average of 21%. To be more explicative, coded data entry refers to the use of coding systems such as the ICD (the WHOs international classification of diseases) that allows storing a disease or a diagnosis as a code rather than a textual description. Furthermore, data transfer via networks involves not only medical data, but also it can be used for administrative purposes.

Greece is slightly below the EU average at 10%, but it is used only by 4% of the GPs. One very important parameter of data exchange is security, since important, personal patient data are been transmitted and stored electronically. There is a general pattern that involves the use of passwords. In the EU27 94% use password protected access, however Greece with a 59% use of password protection has one of the lowest rates in Europe. There are several other methods, such as encryption and the use of electronic signatures, that require not only a dedicated infrastructure but must also be present at both ends—issues that makes them harder to use and more rarely used in the EU.

The use of computer during consultation (display a patients file, supportive information, better explanation of medical issues by means of photos, graphs,etc.) is one more very important feature. In Greece, 30% takes advantage of such a feature, while the EU average is around 66%, although one out of two GP practices is equipped with a computer.

It is worth mentioning that in general there is a very positive attitude towards ICT, its importance and role in the improvement of the quality of health care systems. That positive attitude seems to be independent on whether a country is more of an eHealth laggard or a frontrunner.

The citizens' perspective

It is common knowledge amongst European countries that there is a high doctor-to-patient ratio in Greece, which makes personal contact with health professional the first source of information for the patients. Unfortunately, as mentioned earlier, not only is there a digital divide in Greece, but there is also a gap in the health services provided to rural areas and islands—especially in the winter months.

The perception of the Internet in Greece as a source of information for H&I is positive, given that awareness about Internet services and eHealth in general is low. Even though, the results of the eHealth trends survey indicate resistance to innovative eHealth technologies, people in Greece welcome the opportunity to access their EHR online, and that is a starting point for promoting the use of the Internet for H&I and, in the long term, eHealth.

Awareness activities are necessary for the citizens to recognize the benefits and establish a favorable image for eHealth. This is the only way to ease social inequalities and support the re-engineering of the health care sector providing high quality, affordable, and accessible health care to the citizens and visitors of Greece, even in the remote rural areas and the isolated islands of Aegean Sea.[2]

Indicative best practices
♦ eHealth Unit at Sotiria Hospital

The eHealth Unit at Sotiria Hospital[3] incorporated ICT into its clinical practice in 1999 to help a largely elderly and socially disadvantaged community. Since its inception, the programme has evolved to include home and community-based health and social care solutions that use e-health technologies to manage chronic long term illnesses.

♦ Health-e-Child

The Health-e-Child project[4] aims at developing an integrated healthcare platform for European pediatrics, providing seamless integration of traditional and emerging sources of biomedical information. The long-term goal of the project is to provide uninhibited access to universal biomedical knowledge repositories for personalized and preventive healthcare, large-scale information-based biomedical research and training, and informed policy making.

♦ Integrated pre-hospital health emergency services in the Crete region

An integrated pre-hospital health emergency management system was developed to support optimal response management of pre-hospital health emergencies.[5]

♦ Cardio Express telemedical services

Cardio Express telemedicine services is a company that operates a modern call and control centre with the aim of providing instant evaluation on a case-by-case basis and suggesting the best available treatment options. An experienced team of eight cardiologists responds to patients' calls and analyse the available clinical information and symptoms provided by the patient or by his EHR. In the case of a cardiological problem that could be treated through self-management, an appropriate care plan is defined, including the required medication.

Conclusion
Greece is a particularly interesting case for the eHealth trends survey due to the low penetration of the Internet. eHealth in Greece appears to be by large a grass root phenomenon that has emerged within a mere 4- to 10-year period and is not the result of any planned action from the health care authorities. Although the population in Greece but also Europe has never been healthier,

health care systems are scrambling to effectively cope with costs and demand. In the meantime, there is little knowledge on how eHealth will influence health care delivery.

Perception and use of the Internet assert the existence of a wide digital divide in Greece. However, favorable disposition towards online EHR access and hesitance towards telemedicine suggest that this divide can be bridged with education, user-oriented services, and incentives.

DR. KORINNA ZOI KARAMAGKIOLI is currently serving as Resident in Nuclear medicine at the Alexandra University Hospital- Athens, Greece. Previous working experience includes a one-year residency in Nuclear medicine and Clinical Physiology in the Department of Clinical Physiology at the Central Hospital of Karlstad, Sweden. She has also for worked as District Doctor in the Public Medical Center of Loutraki, a 5,000 habitants region in South Greece. Dr. Karamagkioli was awarded from the President of the Greek Red Cross, for the voluntary service as trainer in the First Aid seminars organized by the Greek Red Cross (March-April 2005). She also offers voluntary services (participates part in missions, training programmes) with the "Medicines du Monde-Greece." Dr. Karamagkioli is Member of the following professionals organizations: Athens Medical Association (Registry No 060534) Swedish National board of Health and Welfare-Socialstyrelsen, General Medical Council (UK), Greek Medicines Du Monde, European Association of Nuclear Medicine and European Association of Radiology.

ENDNOTES

1. http://www.observatory.gr/page/default.asp?la=1&id=2101&pk=400&return=183

2. eHealth Consumer Trends Survey in Greece: Results of the 1st phase. FORTH-ICS TR-365, December 2005. (Updated July 2006) http://www.ics.forth.gr/ftp/tech-reports/2006/2006.TR365_eHealth_Consumer_Trends_Survey.pdf

3. http://www.epractice.eu/cases/Sotiriatelecare

4. http://www.epractice.eu/cases/HeC

5. eHealth in Action – Good Practice in European Countries http://www.epractice.eu/document/5477

References

Doupi P, eHealth strategy and implementation. Activities in GREECE. Report in the framework of the eHealth ERA project. STAKES April 2007

Chronaki C.E, Kouroubali A, et all eHealth Consumer Trends Survey in Greece: Results of the 1st phase. FORTH-ICS TR-365, December 2005. (Updated July 2006)

Health, Health Care and Welfare in Greece, Hellenic Republic, Ministry of Health and Welfare, January 2003.

Snapshots of Health Systems, Susanne Grosse-Tebbe, Josep Figueras (Editors). Greece (p.24-26). European Observatory on Health Systems and Policies, 2004.

Study on the use of ICT in the health area. Report from the Hellenic observatory of information society, 2008. http://www.observatory.gr/page/default.asp?la=1&id=2101&pk=400&return=183

Case of Sotiria Hospital eHealth Unit, available at: http://www.epractice.eu/cases/Sotiriatelecare

Case of ehealth child, available at: http://www.epractice.eu/cases/HeC

eHealth in Action—Good Practice in European Countries http://www.epractice.eu/document/5477

eUser project: eHealth Country Report for Greece. Available online at URL: http://www.euser-eu.org/ShowCase.asp?CaseTitleID=570&CaseID=1207&IDFocus0=3

Chapter 9

Working Criteria in the Management of E-Health Projects

Mario Po'

It is not so much expert knowledge, which I have not, as the experience in the creation of digital healthcare systems, together with the executive planning and implementation of the National Health Care Unit of Asolo, Italy, (http://www.ulssasolo.ven.it) that allows me to suggest some working criteria for the management of e-health solutions.

1ST CRITERION: Does digital technology applied to health care produce savings or costs?

There are no widespread experiences and readily available reliable data showing that technological innovations applied to medical activities actually reduces management costs or lead to decreased investments. The claims to the contrary most often heard overlook the fact that at least every introduction of new technology impacts with important organizational variables. The old organization, the previous professional culture, the persistent managerial constraints, almost always coexist with the new organizational expressions required by the investments being made, thus creating a "productive factor" not easy to chuck out, and that, in the meantime, weighs down the income statement. An interesting example is the consumption of paper, which has not dropped in these recent years of significant dematerialisation of services and is accompanied by substantial investments for printers for desk-top computers. But why do we still need printers in a dematerialised workflow? Why store hard copy of files?

In short, the combination of "old" and "new" systems involves costs that are not so transitory. This is an objective reason that explains the difficulty of achieving "savings" in the short/medium term, i.e., the period of time while the previous organizational characteristics are gradually being replaced by the new ones.

It might, therefore, be believed that better economic performances could be obtained over a longer period of time. But in the long run, technology itself will offer new solutions that will make the earlier solutions obsolescent. Therefore, the process will start all over again, if not from stage one, at least from a level in which new investments will require a new economic framework within the same clinical-managerial scope, or in a contiguous area, while at the same time failing to compensate the higher costs involved and demeaning the value of the alleged "savings" previously achieved.

There are numerous instances proving these failed economic expectations: the introduction of filmless radiology, the advent of email, online reservations, e-prescribing, etc.

However, all of the above is not an argument against technological innovation; the benefits in terms of health care for the population as well as professional activity of the operators are formidable enough to justify such choices. Technology has no need to "apologize" for promising to deliver improbable savings. Clinical ICT systems are so important, sometimes indispensable, that they are "justified" by the operational and functional opportunities they can offer. Even more so, the virtual benefits obtainable from any investment in this field ensure a quick payback for the investment (see Table 1). But this is an eminently technical issue.

Table 1. *Estimated current value of annual costs and benefits of e-Health for a virtual health care economy.*

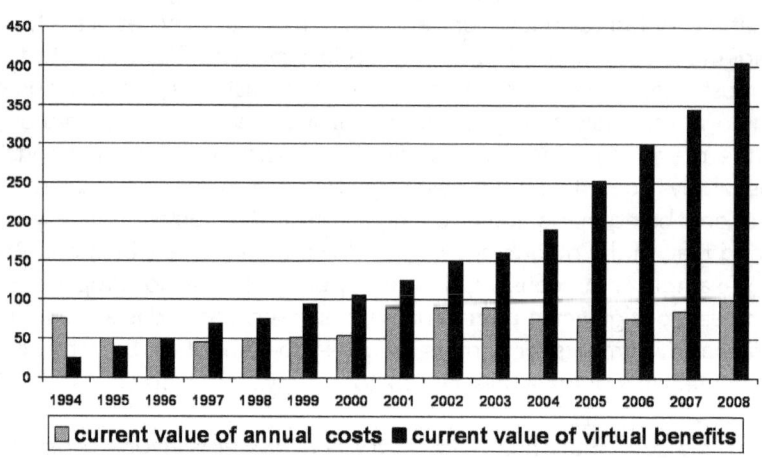

current value of annual costs ■ current value of virtual benefits

Data font:Assinform, 2009

2ND CRITERION: ICT technology is never wrong (even though it is not necessarily right).

The importance of organizational variables in a health facility should be taken into account also when considering the implementation complexities in introducing ICT solutions in hospitals.

The presence of numerous areas of expertise, the different job profiles, the widely varying and constantly evolving operative techniques, the working connections outside the main application context, all offer reasons that explain the difficult identification of responsibilities and areas of competence within an e-health project. Within this "natural" technical executive criticality, the technology being introduced is often indiscriminately blamed for otherwise endemic gaps, delays, mismatches, etc.

These behaviors are sometimes more of a cultural attitude than a technical stand, and therefore, apparently harmless because barely perceptible. Yet, it is of great importance to nip them in the bud, because confusion in management planning can also result in confusion in solutions, time, costs, etc. We cannot always expect formal diagnoses of an impasse in the implementation of the project, or self-criticism regarding the willingness to join the project or open criticism of the significant contents of the ICT investment. The hospital organization is well adept at hiding their reluctance to change and can exploit the possibility to use indisputable clinical priorities, lingo technicalities and all that is within the arsenal of the medical profession to shift the problems associated with technical implementations away from themselves and solely towards the technology.

However, it is the organization that plans the introduction of a new ICT intervention; and it is within the organization that the problems subject to change are created. And it is once again the organization that establishes rules for the technology.

Table 2. *When Organization and technology are winning factors.*

Tecnology wins

Compromise area	Success area
Organization loses	Organization wins
Loss area	Compromise area

Technology loses

So, emphasizing this conviction, we can say that the main responsibilities and tasks in the subsequent stages of the project almost always lie with those in charge of the organizational fields.

In project management, there are, therefore, areas of failure, compromise, and success attributable to technology and conditioned by the mode and extent of the cooperation established between the two factors. This interrelationship cannot be a clash or even an area of suspicion, and instead must be virtuously cultivated in order to bring the whole system to yield the best possible results in the shortest time possible.

3RD CRITERION: Working with the integration of homogeneous digital systems, and even more so with heterogeneous systems, means reaping benefits and opportunities "naturally."

A hospital operating system is by definition an integrated system from a clinical, organizational, and technological point of view. There is abundant literature on the subject of malpractice resulting from failing to see the patient's clinical reality as an integrated system, because the person being treated is the model par excellence of the integration of apparatuses, organs, physiology and, why not, emotions.

This objective data must be the driving force to organize integrated healthcare digital systems capable of accommodating all the work areas existing within the hospital simultaneously and consistently.

If this integration is not a native feature of a system, it must then be achieved through later integration processes. This can be accomplished in several stages within a given time (preferably short to medium), so as to make the benefits of such integration clear, as long as the process and the arrival point are clear as well. Like, for example, in public access services to hospital activities.

In these cases, technology is very helpful to avoid interruptions in the operational flow, allowing the patient to "be taken in charge" by the attending physician, with the preparation of an e-prescription for referral to specialist care, and then guided by the ICT system logically and continuously to book specialist treatment, pay the ticket cost, where applicable, get the specialist service required, and finally, get the clinical report. All this is done without having to register the patient's access or his/her treatment at any later administrative-clinical stage after the initial booking; without producing repetitive paperwork; without having to verify the correspondence of the data in relation to the person treated; without forcing the attending physician to wait for the physical delivery of the test results.

Integrating heterogeneous systems first of all means connecting different healthcare and administration software. In this way, the benefits are measurable also in terms of managerial opportunities acquired by the hospital, which will enable to understand and measure goals and performances that would otherwise be excluded from any evaluation scheme.

The heterogeneity of the contents of the activities of the departments "naturally" participating in a clinical document flow should not be a hindrance to the need to treat as a digital integrated flux (see Table 3) any pre-existing effort in this direction.

Table 3. *Clinical digital documental flow.*

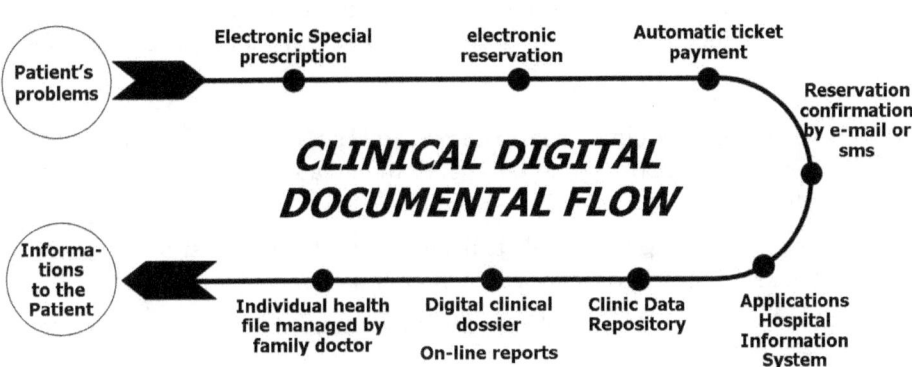

It is a claim that must be reaffirmed. Job opportunities for healthcare and health service professionals are so high that there is no reason why a non-clinical software should not transfer its data into a document management system or why the software managing patients' access to hospital services should be limited to organizing only the entry-level stage of hospital admittances, or why the administrative-economic part should be a separate system even though it derives its information from clinical events.

Each clinical need of the patient has an information content regarding the patient. The subject is always the same. The solution, therefore, must be integration.

4TH CRITERION: A digital clinical system cannot be maintained without a patient-oriented documental solution.

A health care software is required to fulfill two main functions: an internal function for the management of diagnostics and curative treatments; an external function to provide patients with the information that will make them autonomous in the knowledge of their clinical situation. When this dual concept fails, the system is not working with the potential and convenience for which it was designed.

If application is restricted to the first area, benefits will be severely limited, because as a result they will be achieved only within the scope of "clinical production," no matter how technically and ethically important that may be. For example, it is unthinkable that a PACS (Picture Archiving and Communication System) system should not also be the source for an application that provides document to private end users. It should become the core of a "clinical safe" fed by the medical activities, managing to justify costly investments because of its important spin-off effects in terms of quantity and quality of services available to a large number of people.

However, this external strategic function must be accompanied by the resolution to embrace definite working criteria, including methodological ones, such as:

1. The project should be set up immediately so that the results achieved can soon be translated into benefits immediately seen and felt by the citizenry;

2. The whole hospital and all its health care satellites must operate with the same standards, applicable in all situations of intervention;

3. The internal and external ICT network must be adequately resourced and sized;

4. Health care ICT applications should be integrable (if they are not already part of a single integrated environment);

5. Implementation must be supported by a training program for operators and a communication strategy for dissemination to the public.

A significant example of good implementation of a clinical system is the choice of National Healthcare Unit ULSS 8 Asolo (Italy) to make the largest number of services immediately available to the public, including those which, although unseen by the patient, are an expression of a documental version of a clinical management system. The service is accessible through their website (http://www.ulssasolo.ven.it): data goes from Radiology PACS into the electronic medical records; from Test Laboratory LIS into the electronic medical records; from the Cardiology CIS into the electronic medical records, etc.

Through the website of the Health Care Unit, citizens have access to the clinical information they require, in a networking logic in which they are increasingly active and independent.

Table 4. *ULSS 8 web site.*

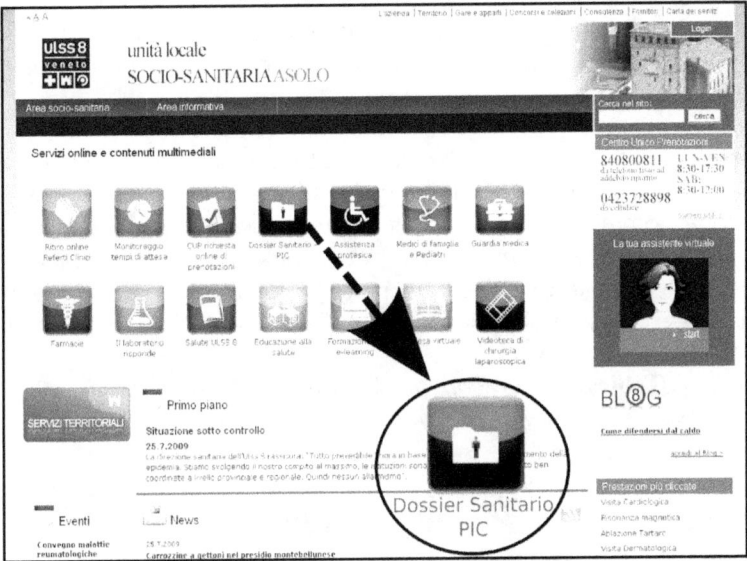

5TH CRITERION: Individual operative defections are not acceptable from operative teams.

Hospital activities should offer all users the same performance, i.e., the same clinical standard of diagnosis, treatment and information. This means that the operational indicators provided by an HIT service should be ensured at all times and in all cases, with the ensuing inevitable commitment by the medical and technical components of the clinical team to operate following the same criteria.

When, even if only occasionally, a member of the group fails to comply with one of the procedural stages (e.g., uploading data into system, recording a performance, omitting the digital signature on the report, etc.) the system loses its foremost characteristic, i.e., continuity, thereby losing credibility as well. The impression given will be of occasional data input, which prevents the formation of complete individual medical records and, above all, this will give rise to doubts on the availability of specific data in the future.

Furthermore, it should be noted that the benefits of HIT services are not linked to individual exploits but to constant and consistent behaviors, always complying with the same rules (very probably banal, and perhaps even indispensably repetitive, but essential).

It is, therefore, necessary that every electronic innovation, especially in online services to citizens, should be based on the prior and supportive participation to the project by the professionals who provide the services. The support must be a constant in the operation of the service, and continuously monitored and sustained.

There are several ways to give that support to the members of a team. Experience shows two. The first is highlighting the effects for better performance in the professional commitment of clinicians and technicians; the second is financially encouraging the achievement of individual targets in a finalized, objectively verifiable way (see Table 5 for the percentage of family doctors using e-prescriptions, in the experience of National Health Care Unit ULSS. 8 Asolo, Italy).

Table 5. *ULSS 8, day-to-day transmission of electronic special prescriptions by family doctors.*

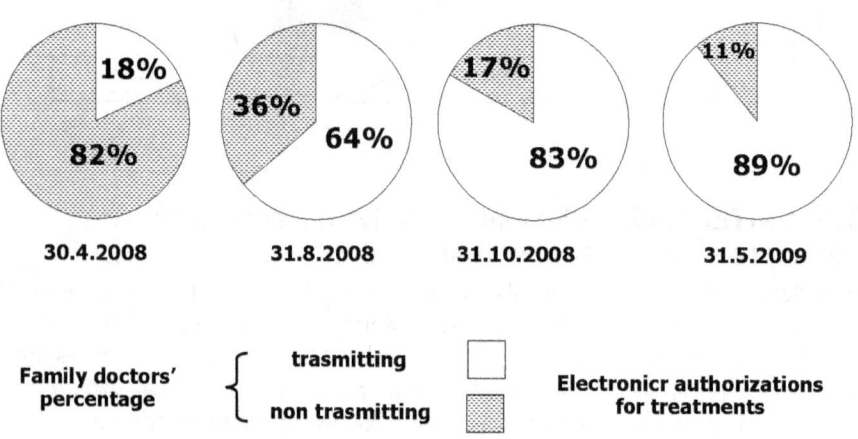

6TH CRITERION: In conducting an ICT project, attach excessive importance to one particular element; it is a much less decisive factor than the organization would have you believe.

When planning an e-health project it is almost inevitable that the various "stakeholders" will raise issues on subjects that may apparently sound decisive for the continued implementation of the project while actually being of secondary importance. The complaints about these issues sometimes respond to a logic of verification of the soundness of the project on the part of those who are less convinced of the value of the process or, less maliciously, it is raised by the exaggerated concerns of technical specialists who, almost by professional deformation, tend to mistake a "part for the whole."

This observation intends to highlight an issue of great impact for the concreteness and especially for the timeline that a project can take on when proceeding from its inception to the implementation stage. For this reason, the working method must favour a rapid pace, where "fast and rough" is better than "slow and elegant," in the belief that after having involved all potential stakeholders it is necessary to apply two rules in monitoring the development of an ITC project for heath care facilities:

1. If the first attempt fails, try and try again, but only within a given time frame;

2. In a process, any positive result must be achieved within a time frame of days.

Failing to follow these rules would mean realizing only too late that one has continued to work along the wrong track while there were sufficiently clear signals right from the start showing the validity of the project in relation to its capabilities to achieve the desired overall results.

Therefore, it is not so much the definition or immediate solution of specific issues that warrant the implementation of the project. These issues must indeed be addressed and dealt with, as they represent a huge management cost, but only after the certainty of obtaining a result has been reached.

7TH CRITERION: Geo-medical integration, i.e., the territorial scope of a digital system, maximizes opportunities.

If the integration between clinical systems and different e-gov systems lies at the basis of the important opportunities made available to patients and operators, greater benefits can be obtained if the integration is applied on a larger geographical scale. The interconnections created within a single hospital can be repeated also between the various hospitals in a city, region, and nationwide network, achieving extraordinary results in terms of completeness of clinical knowledge of the inhabitants of that area, the immediacy of a detailed intervention method in emergency situations, the possibility of having the clinical results obtained at different times interact using different technologies, more or less simple or sophisticated methods, etc.

An example of the potential inherent in a solution of geo-medical integration can be seen in a territorial PACS (whose "catchment area" may be geographically small yet serving several hospitals) that would disengage the citizens of that area from the need to use only the nearest health facility. They could be referred to any of the hospitals in the area (either through ER services or Specialist clinics), which would have access to the same radiological archive, usable by every facility, containing such a large database that radiological reporting would be much more accurate and secure than in many other circumstances.

A similar perspective can easily be realized using the technological systems of other specialist areas such as test laboratories, or Pathology, etc., which use very standardized methods that easily lend themselves to a quasi-modular dissemination over a vast area.

Indeed, these geo-medical solutions imply a significant simplification of the actual medical record processing, as this instrument would directly receive its contents from clinical and health care services, which, in a case such as radiology, would have a formidable ally in a picture archiving and communication systems at regional or national level. But the system could be expanded to other areas of specialist health care.

Yet this technological formula is essentially unknown in hospitals, which work with self-contained peripheral solutions. We still have to deal with a patchy presence of PACS in hospitals (see Italian situation in the following tables). Is it more expensive, at this point, to allocate funding for other hospital PACS systems, or for territorial systems at regional or sub-regional level, or at least at the level of each single National Health Care Unit?

Table 6. *Hospital supported by RIS/PACS technology (analysis on 672 Italian hospitals).*

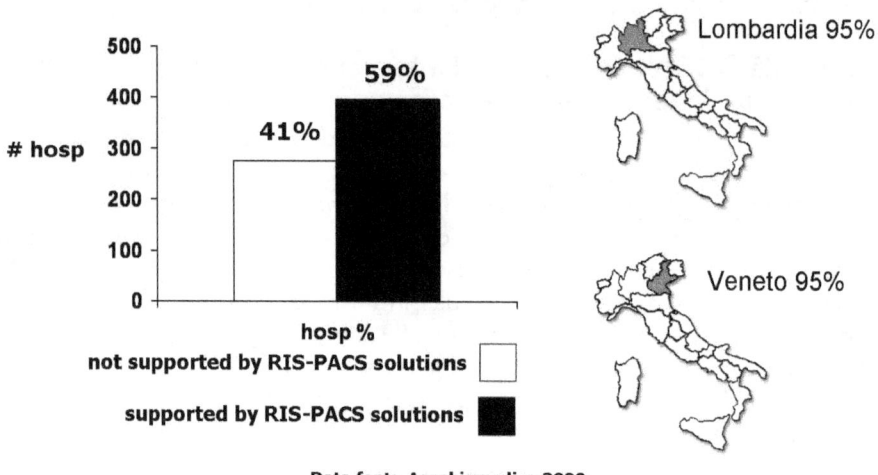

Data font: Assobiomedica 2008

8TH CRITERION: Web 2.0 is not an instrument of therapeutic and diagnostic co-management.

Health care services shaped by web 2.0 logic are becoming increasingly frequent. It is a logic different from that of "traditional" ICT applications; it also differs in the relationships between the various actors in the health care chain from anything we have known so far. Not only because of the content of information that it should develop between networkers, but especially because of their role.

The patients cease to be only the recipient of health care and research because they become part of a virtual community and stand on an equal footing (but sometimes also with the role of experts) with other patients, doctors, specialists and researchers, in producing therapeutic interventions, psychological support, behaviour protocols, classifications within a case series, etc.

Web 2.0 has thus radically changed the way of planning e-health. Citizens and patients have never had such a pivotal role before. It is an unprecedented challenge for health systems and hospital organizations, which tend to be schematic and hierarchical realities, especially in the ownership of knowledge (real or presumed).

This new logic leads to two practical consequences in digital planning:

1. A complete replacement of many ICT solutions in operation today (which are now obsolete in their philosophy of the passivity of the patient), thus giving way to a broad spectrum of radically new interventions;

2. an evolutionary development of solutions with a solidly "good" core based on the subjectivity of the patient (or, in any case, where the patient was the reason for the project), but whose technology must now be refocused.

As always, however, we must have a clear idea of the mission that we attach to Web 2.0 design, or, better still, to Medicine 2.0. We are not confronted with a scenario of "patients" that are virtually autonomous and pro-active in their diagnosis and treatment. Nor can we hope a situation of co-managing the doctor-patient relationship, which would lead to conflict and serious risks. Instead, we might think that the dissemination of the instruments of knowledge will leave a share of information to the patients so that they can become one of the prime movers in health care, not just passive recipients.

On-line access to their data and clinical records, multimedia services, SMS services, on-line booking operations, community activities such as chat, forums, blogs, wikis, etc., can greatly improve communications, health care information, the relationship with the patients and their autonomy, but they are not new treatment methods.

The effectiveness of these ICT tools in health care has not been fully evaluated yet, but there are all the prerequisites needed to rewrite the rules of the physician-patient and patient–hospital relationships.

These new rules (which are basically those of the first world wide web: allow people to collaborate) must inform all health care ICT project developments, which will prove convincing, today more than yesterday, if they can give positive answers to these questions:

1. Will the e-health project ensure direct informational benefits to the patient?
2. Will these benefits be achievable in the short term?
3. Will they be permanent?

Promoting the autonomy of the individual in health care has always been, after all, the reason for a good system. That is why, today, with Medicine 2.0 the response to these needs is just a click away.

Table 7. *The reasons for clicking: Seeking medical information.*

36%	**Learn** what other people think of a pharmaceutical drug or treatment		**14%**	**Share** experiences and information about a pharmaceutical drug or treatment
31%	**Search** other patients' experiences		**13%**	**Seek** users' opinions and suggestions on a hospital
27%	**Get** information to manage one's disease		**10%**	**Seek** users' opinions and suggestions on a physician
17%	**Receive** emotional support		**8%**	**Feel part** of a community
14%	**Share** experiences and information about a disease		**100%**	**TOTAL**

Source: Juniter Research 2007

MARIO PO' is Executive Director of Health Local Authority (ULSS n. 8) of Asolo. He coordinated the planning the realization of the ICT Plan strategic as well as the implementation of the Service Centre for the logistic of the drugs and the Digital Warehouse. He coordinated also the new management system of e-learning and the first Italian Network of e-learning. He guides, at last, the business plan on the e-health multimedia education. Previously in the ULSS of Treviso, he took care of a public-private partnership for the management of Rehabilitative Hospital of Motta di Livenza. In the Veneto Region, he was deputy for international regional relationships in Alpe Adria's and Central-East Europe area. Then, in the Minister of Transports' Cabinet in Rome, he was charged of activities connected to the international relations for the area of the European Union and Mediterranean.

REFERENCES

Schael T. (2009), *Sanità elettronica e servizi digitali al cittadino*, in Voice com news, anno X – 02.2009, Italia.

Francesconi A. (2008), *"Dangerous liaisons": manager, professionisti e tecnologie. Il caso delle aziende sanitarie*, Università Ca' Foscari di Venezia; Venezia.

Bryan S., Weatherburn T.D.C., Watkins J.R., Buxon M.J. (1999), *The benefits of hospital-wide PACS: a survey of clinical users of radiology services*, in "Br. J. Radiol.", Vol. 72, 469-472.

Cicchetti A. (2004), *La progettazione organizzativa. Principi strumenti e applicazioni nelle organizzazioni sanitarie*, FrancoAngeli, Milano.

Cox B, Dawe N. (2002), *Evaluation of the impact of a PACS system on an intensive care unit*, in "Journal of management in Medicine", voi. 16(2/3), pp. 199-205.

Francesconi A. (2007), *Innovazione organizzativa e tecnologica in sanità. Il ruolo dell'health technology assessment*, FrancoAngeii, Milano.

Giribona P. (1989), *Principles for PACS evaluation*, European Community workshop on PACS, Avelro, Portugal.

Kissick W. (1994), *Medicines Dilemmas: Infinite needs versus finite resources*, Yale University Press, New Heven and London.

Maggi B. (1989), *L'organizzazione dei servizi sanitari, in "Sviluppo e Organizzazione"*, Vol. 115, 53-64.

Margolin K. (2001), *Web technology and its relevance to PACS and teleradiology—Take II*, in "Applied Radiology", Vol. 30(2), 28-32.

Munch H., Engelmann U., Schroeter A., Meinzer H.P. (2003), *Web-based distribution of radiological images from PACS to EPR*, in "International Congress Series", Vol. 1256, 873-879.

Orlikowski W.J. (1992), *The duality of technology: Rethinking the concept of technology in organizations*, in "Organization Science", Vol. 3(3), 398-427.

Ravagnani R. (2000), *Information technology e gestione del cambiamento organizzativo*, Egea, Milano.

Scott W.R., Reuf M., Mendel P.J., Caronna C.A. (2000), *Institutional change and healthcare organizations*, The University of Chicago Press, Chicago.

Thompson T.G., Brailer D.J. (2004), *The Decade of Health Information Technology: Delivering Consumer-centric and Information-rich Health Care. Framework for Strategic Action*, Office of the Secretary, National Coordinator for Health Information Technology, U.S. Department of Health and Human Services, Bethesda, MD.

Weick K.E. (1990), *Technology as Equivoque*, in Goodman P.S., Sproull L.S. and Associates (eds.), *Technology and organizations*, Jossey-Bass, San Fransisco, CA.

Chapter 10

Toward Sustainable Health— What is Missing From an IT Perspective?

Octavian Purcarea, M.D., Global Solution Manager, Worldwide Health, Microsoft

In 2004, countries around the world spent a total of $4.1 trillion (USD) on health care. Among member countries of the Organization for Economic Cooperation and Development (OECD), governments and citizens spent an average of 11 percent of GDP on health.[1] Healthcare spending in the United States alone reached $2 trillion by 2006, consuming 16 percent of the country's GDP—and for all that, it only ranks 72nd among OECD countries in quality of care.

Worldwide, today, there are 260 million elders; 1 billion citizens are overweight; 860 million patients suffer from some type of chronic disease; 75-85 percent of all spending on health care targets chronic diseases; and globally there are only 18 million hospital beds in 200,000 hospitals to treat the sick and wounded. An ever-increasing shortage of doctors and nurses, and skilled ancillary personnel, magnify the increasing demand by citizens for healthcare services. As populations in developed nations age and the impact of public health issues such as smoking, obesity, poor diet and lack of exercise grows, these costs will continue to rise—placing a significant burden on governments who provide health care for their citizens as well as employers who provide it for their workers. A rising percentage of healthcare budgets are being spent on the management of chronic or long-term conditions such as Diabetes, COPD, and Cardiovascular diseases. Estimates from the International Diabetes Foundation are that costs from this single chronic condition could overwhelm most public healthcare systems by 2025.

Many of these growing costs come from challenges in managing vast amounts of health information. Healthcare has long been an information-driven industry—we're all familiar with the image of a doctor making rounds with her clipboard—but software has not kept up with the deluge of data that healthcare providers now struggle with. Important patient information lives in too many different "silos," locked into systems that cannot easily communicate with each other. Too much information is still captured on paper and dumped into filing cabinets. To get a complete picture of patients' health—and to make sound medical decisions—healthcare providers must synthesize information from many different sources, meaning everything from X-rays and health records to EKGs, MRIs and CT scans. This is fast becoming an excessive burden.

Though new diagnostic modalities and new medication discoveries are occurring daily, the delivery of healthcare has not changed in a significant way in more than 50 years. The industry delivers care in a way that is still largely manual and paper-based. As there is an increased need to share clinical data in order to track new diseases, coordinated public health infrastructures will become more critical than ever.

Escalating costs; an inconsistent quality of outcomes and therapies; an aging population; clinical research that does not find its way into the mainstream of medical practice for up to a decade on average; rampant inefficiencies caused by a lack of readily available clinical information causing redundancy in diagnostics; inappropriate hospitalizations; medication errors; and preventable deaths—all of these plague the global health industry. Despite significant differences in the delivery structure and payment methods for health care, the issues from healthcare customers are remarkably uniform. The need to improve patient safety, contain the spiraling increases in healthcare costs, and match the expectation levels of the citizen living in a connected and digital age are coming together in the perfect storm of challenges for healthcare providers and governments funding health delivery.

Empowering *clinicians* to work more efficiently and effectively in the "digital work style" of the new world of healthcare work should be at the center of any healthcare delivery organization's strategy as it addresses the coming era of rapid change and increasing global integration. Some clinicians claim that they need for a "GPS system for clinical practice:" something that helps them navigate through the massive amount of information and alerts them to what is important and what is not important, what needs to be done now and what can wait, and provides a more global view of what is occurring in the population of patients under their care.

As we move toward a world of healthcare that must become more fluid, less centralized and less certain about old assumptions and old models, Information Technology is evolving in ways that will empower providers, teams and individual citizens to realize their potential in a new world of healthcare work.

A wealth of studies support the premise that connecting people, systems, and services is vital for the provision of good healthcare in the world, and contributes significantly to the establishment and functioning of the global market by ensuring the free flow of eHealth products and services.[2]

The advance of eHealth applications and services and the wider level of implementation in the world oblige policy makers, industry, the medical profession and other stakeholders to carefully assess future developments, taking into account the need to build seamless information networks across borders in regions and countries. eHealth has the potential to enable adequate support to any defined health policy regarding citizen, care delivery or managerial needs.

Additionally, eHealth offers the citizen important opportunities for improved access to better health systems; eHealth is expected to boost the quality and effectiveness of the services offered; eHealth has also the potential to empower citizens in dealing with their own health.

Through the seamless transmission of information related to health issues and also on the managerial level, eHealth will contribute to an increased quality and efficiency of health services; eHealth will also provide an opportunity for economic benefits; it will contribute to major cost savings in the delivery of high quality and effective health services.

Subsequently, eHealth creates a major business potential for industry; however, further market acceptance and trust in health services will depend on interoperability of the services and applications. Interoperability is a key issue to the faster adoption of ICT throughout the healthcare systems all over the world.

eHealth can provide a unique set of tools for overcoming many of the challenges that health delivery systems are facing today and developing new patient-centred health systems that meet the complex needs of our changing world. Hard evidence proves that eHealth is already providing real benefits to people as well as real savings in public expenditure.[3] In the Health domain, the eHealth industry is one of the largest growing sectors with a double digit annual growth and an estimated size of 20 Billion Euro in 2006, forecast to become 50 Billion Euro by 2010.

eHealth has been identified as a "lead market" in Europe that can contribute substantially to both societal and economic progress, a major element in the European Council's agreed Innovation policy document "Creating an Innovative Europe" (Jan 2006).

eHealth will help individuals in general, and elderly people in particular, to live independently for longer. eHealth could allow to treat up to 40% of all the emergency care cases treated in hospitals.

Through the careful choice of eHealth applications, we can contribute to the care of the many chronic illnesses that individuals experience, especially as they grow older. It is known that *"Chronic diseases, such as heart disease, stroke, cancer, chronic respiratory diseases and diabetes, are by far the leading cause of mortality in the world, representing 60% of all deaths. Out of the 35 million people who died from chronic disease in 2005, half were under 70 and half were women."* [4]

We can be successful in achieving better prevention and prediction in healthcare, greater personalization of healthcare processes and, ultimately, more productivity and economic benefits in the achievement of good health for world people. Placing more emphasis on the key elements of prevention, better chronic disease management, patient and citizen empowerment, and the health and ICT education of patients is an area of untapped potential.

However, the potential of eHealth is far from being achieved. There are important challenges related to usability of eHealth tools and trust in the organizational model around use of these tools. In order to achieve an efficient and **sustainable** management of chronic diseases that are the main source of spending in developed countries, one should think that two of the most important barriers are the **trust and usability.** Let's take a closer look.

Usability has been one of the major causes of failures in the IT programs; with a poor design, the health professionals lose time, can add other errors of interpretation and finally abandon the use of the software.

Several studies have shown that due to the low usability, many IT programs are abandoned. For example, a Belgian study from 2004 showed that for from large population of General Practitioners and more than 133.000 contact with the patient, the Electronic Patient Record was underused, with only 6.7 % of the contact recorded. In Germany, a study performed in 2006 on 72 network of care and 17 from Switzerland, showed that only 20% of the care networks have electronic data exchange, only 9% have structured data and only 3% can document the care processes electronically.[5]

How can an IT application become acceptable by the health professionals? The IT industry must take a particular care on these aspects. Microsoft issued the Common User Interface[6] guidelines as a result of a project funded by the UK NHS. As a formal definition, the Microsoft Health Common User Interface (CUI) provides User Interface Design Guidance and Toolkit controls that address a wide range of patient safety concerns for healthcare organizations worldwide, enabling a new generation of safer, more usable and compelling health applications to be quickly and easily created.

Moreover, the software vendors have left all the technical complexity for the user, as the Tesler's[7] Law of Conservation of Complexity is suggesting: "Every application has an inherent amount of irreducible complexity. The only question is who will have to deal with it—the user, the application developer, or the platform developer?"

What would be the solution? The only way to get to the desired level of usability is to design software that would reflect the work process of the user (workflow) and the mental model (concepts) of the user (terminology). Such a development would give birth to a new generation of Clinical information systems (partner level) that would enable assisted clinical decision, use of care path and real disease management (built on evidence based medicine and evidence based management).

Figure 1.

1. Software behavior should reflect the work process of the user (workflow)

2. Software objects should reflect the mental model (concepts) of the user (terminology)

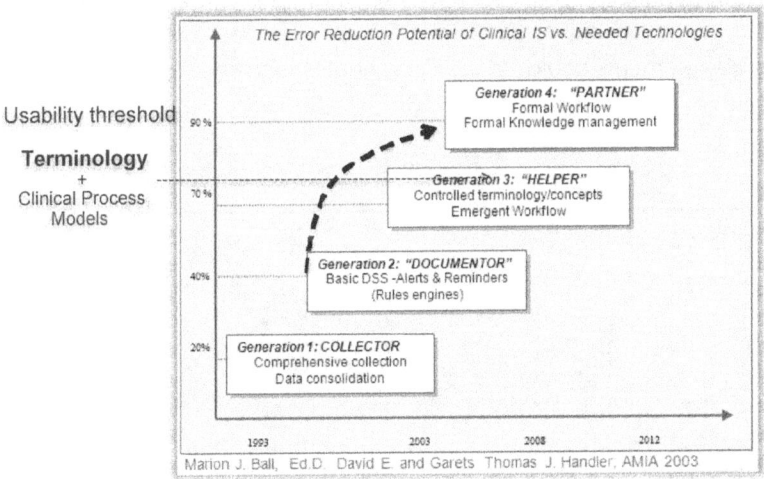

This kind of innovative software is developed by some of the vendors (such as Medicognos, C-Systems, Fresenius, Parrot Systems) and is seen as a very promising solution for many IT plans regarding management of chronic diseases in view of a sustainable healthcare. Moreover, innovative data entry, speech recognition, surface computing[8] are some of the innovations able to increase the speed of interaction of health professionals and patients in eHealth.

What about trust? Several IT programs across Europe initiated by the governments and/or insurance companies have encountered resistance from the health professionals. Imagine how difficult it would be to change the behaviors of the health professionals and persuade them to use new IT tools, change the way they are working and communicating. One solution to the **trust problem** would be to allow them to decide on the care path, on the design of the IT tools and to involve them in the overall organization of a chronic disease management program. In exchange, performance and quality management should be enabled so as a program of incentives. There is no other solution to the trust problem than the collaboration, active involvement of the health professionals in any of the insurance and governmental healthcare programs. Patient associations and customer rights association should be deeply involved in large IT programs in order to achieve adherence of the users from the inception of the initiatives.

What about **sustainability**? The paradigm of care versus cure is the one to which we adhere. Considering an individual, a patient as whole, an entity with personality, living in certain environment (social, natural) and having certain genetic predispositions and habits is offering the key to sustainable healthcare. Using the IT tools we can inform, empower, facilitate the information of the patients and enhance communication between caregivers and the patients.

One of the key elements could be the Personnel Health Record supported by a platform such as HealthVault.[9]

Figure 2.

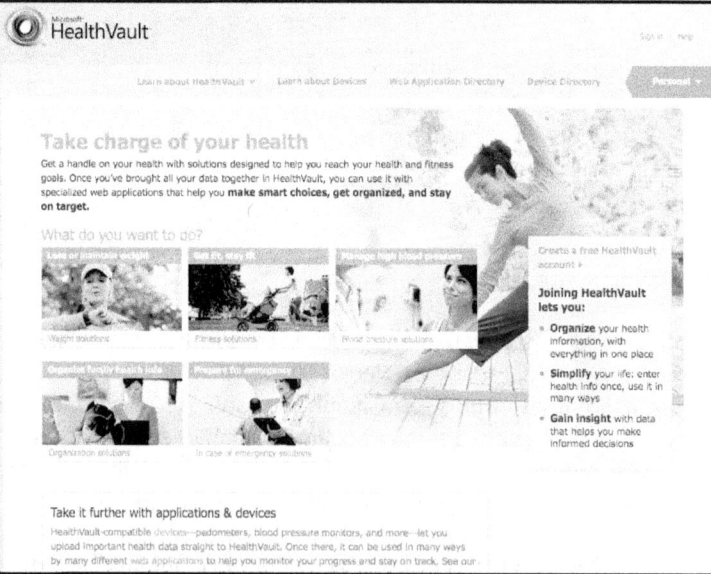

Such solutions could facilitate in Europe the empowerment of individuals and pave the way towards efficient disease management solutions and a real, incentive-based containment of costs.

The IT solutions are available and must be wisely assembled in a comprehensive eHealth solution that will help all the stakeholders (favoring change in behavior, empowering users, increase adherence to the treatment, increase health care user communication and information), while being trusted, usable and sustainable.

The private and public payers should consider a strong involvement of users and other stakeholders in the setting up of adequate governance, planning, design, validation, implementation, evaluation, monitoring, training, information and education, and change management in eHealth implementation.

Establishing **trust** is a major challenge, and this can be addressed by proving the benefits of eHealth through successful pilots, building robust information and training of users. The public powers as well as the private sector should **commit to comply** with the legal framework on data privacy, confidentiality and data security existing in various countries and to various mechanisms for evaluation, monitoring, and education in order to ensure that the patients and health professionals are fully exploiting the potential of their IT tools.

Finally, we strongly believe that there must be a convergence between the solutions in the area of eHealth, eInclusion, eGovernment. This federated approach based on the infrastructure and identification, security, transport, search layers would save costs and allow individuals to take advantage of a wealth of services while using only one ID. Some of these principles have been developed in the Connected Health Platform,10 an open architecture concept developed by Microsoft and accepted by many industry solution vendors.

In conclusion, eHealth will be the tomorrow solution for sustainable healthcare taking into account:

- ♦ Involve users in the design, development and implementation of eHealth tools;
- ♦ Copy the mental model and the usual recommended workflow of health professionals;
- ♦ Create solid proof of concept involving the users;
- ♦ Explore new organizational models and business models based on disease management, network of care and performance indicators;

♦ Empower the individuals, patients, giving them the necessary tools to be informed, monitor their biological parameters and environmental conditions and enhance the communication with the health professionals;

♦ Think in terms of quality management, evidence based medicine coupled with evidence based management, pay per performance and seek for the appropriate IT tools able to deliver such promises;

♦ Take a particular attention to legal framework on data privacy and security of personal information and in order to establish a climate of trust.

OCTAVIAN PURCAREA is a medical doctor with a post-graduate degree in Health Administration (MBA), a general surgery training and more than 10 years of experience in eHealth area. His experience in the private sector in different domains (Health information networks, telemedicine and research in the eHealth area) was followed by six years as Scientific Officer at the European Commission in Directorate General Information Society and Media, for the eHealth Unit. He was in charge with the policy aspects of Interoperability of eHealth applications and the research aspects related to Patient Safety. He joined the Worldwide Health team of Microsoft in 2008 where he is dealing with policy aspects in eHealth, collaboration with international organizations and various communities in eHealth area.

ENDNOTES

1. Ten Statistical Highlights in Global Public Health, World Health Organization, 2007. http://www.who.int/whosis/whostat2007_ 10highlights.pdf

2. The Value Of Health Care Information Exchange And Interoperability: There is a business case to be made for spending money on a fully standardized nationwide system. by Jan Walker, Eric Pan, Douglas Johnston, Julia Adler-Milstein, David W. Bates, and Blackford Middleton—Health Affairs: Web Exclusive, January 19, 2005 (http://content.healthaffairs. org/cgi/reprint/hlthaff.w5.10v1)

2. Wennberg et al. Geography and the Debate Over Medicare Reform, Health Affairs. 02/13/02. W96-W114; Wennberg et al. Use of hospital, physician visits and hospice case during the last six months of like among cohorts loyal to highly respected hospitals in the United States. BMJ. March 13, 2004; Fisher et al. The implications of regional variations in Medicare spending, Part 1: The content, quality and accessibility of care. Annals of Internal Medicine. 2003; 138:273-287; Fisher et al.

The implications of regional variations in Medicare spending, Part 2: The content, quality and accessibility of care. Annals of Internal Medicine. 2003; 138:288-298.

3. See the report eHealth is worth it—http://ec.europa.eu/information_society/newsroom/cf/itemshortdetail.cfm?item_id=2878

4. 2009—World Health Organization http://www.who.int/chp/en/

5. Praxisnetz Studie 2006 Management -Prozesse –Informationstechnologie- Günter Schicker und Oliver Kohlbauer , Wirtschaftsinformatik II Universität Erlangen-Nürnberg

Chapter 11

A Long-term Vision for eHealth— and How to Get It Now

Thaima Samman, Senior Director & Associate General Counsel, Corporate Affairs— Corporate Social Responsibility, Microsoft Europe

Elena Bonfiglioli, Director of Corporate Responsibility for Microsoft Europe, Middle East and Africa

eHealth can improve the delivery of medical care, inspire a shift from cure to prevention, increase efficiency, create new jobs and drive economic growth

Applying technology innovation to healthcare (eHealth) can play a key role in improving the quality and efficiency of medical services by collecting, unlocking and connecting all the information that individuals need to take control of their health and wellness. Like other pivotal breakthroughs in medicine over the past few hundred years, information and communication technology has the potential to revolutionize healthcare and improve the quality of our lives.

Advances in genomics and diagnostic technology are making it easier to spot diseases earlier and treat them more effectively. Machine learning and other techniques adapted from computer science are transforming drug discovery, development and other aspects of medical research, bringing the prospect of life-saving drugs for previously untreatable diseases. And patients are increasingly empowered with technologies that help them cope with chronic conditions and maintain lifelong wellness.

In this article we argue that the technology to realize the vision of tomorrow's healthcare is already available today. In this context we see eHealth as a critical "change agent" helping our societies to make the shift from cure to prevention, from treatment of diseases to a focus on wellness and care.

The benefits arising for individuals, societies, and healthcare systems as a whole from such deep transformation are enormous. We can list them in high-level, broad-brush terms as wider access to healthcare for many more people, lower costs for national systems as well as for hospitals and individuals, better quality of delivery, and economic growth and new jobs.

Microsoft's vision is of a connected healthcare ecosystem that gives patients more control and convenience, better service, and better value; an ecosystem that empowers physicians and providers by giving them the right data in the right format at the right time, enabling them to provide the best treatment and preventive care.

In this article we first outline a long-term vision for technology innovation applied to healthcare. While doing so, we argue that eHealth is more than the digitalisation of traditional healthcare practices. It is about moving healthcare practices on to a new frontier: to improve quality of care, to anticipate rather than cure, and to empower patients to manage their health and remain more independent at home, while at the same time reducing hospitalisation costs.

No wonder, then, that in the U.S., President Barack Obama has argued that eHealth is central not only to healthcare reform, but also to economic renewal. In Europe, both at EU level and in Member States, there is a growing appreciation of how information and communication technology (ICT) can improve the delivery of health services and serve as the glue to hold together an array of medical technologies, improving care while curbing costs.

Alongside the benefits—which illustrate why there is reason to be optimistic about the future of our healthcare systems—this article also acknowledges the risk of the vicious circle of technical and cultural obstacles that must be tackled before eHealth benefits can be realised in Europe. The strong political leadership demonstrated both at EU and national levels will be ever-more needed in the years to come to stimulate the next phase of transformation and innovation in healthcare and realise the promise of eHealth.

Deep partnerships between all stakeholders are needed to move things in the right direction and at the right speed. There is a need for education, innovation and collaboration. Citizens, healthcare consumers, medical professionals and healthcare organizations have a unique opportunity to encourage innovation in eHealth—not by mandating specific technologies or development models, but by setting objective goals and criteria.

When considering technology frameworks and enabling conditions, we look to public authorities to establish a technology framework based on objective, neutral criteria and then encourage all companies to compete. Reward systems should be in place for innovative doctors who make the Internet the foundation of the patient-physician connection and help drive the transformation forward. Physicians should also be encouraged to embrace basic Internet technologies that allow them to communicate more effectively and consistently with patients.

The future is a scalable, patient-centric eHealth System in which, instead of allowing healthcare professionals to control the patient experience and healthcare facilities to control patient records, individuals can take greater responsibility for their overall health and wellness.

Once the basic frameworks and standards are in place, the private sector will be enabled to develop an information infrastructure that connects data, systems, and people. A system that is flexible, interoperable, scalable, private, and secure will ensure that data flows freely and is reused.

The long-term vision and the promise of eHealth: A patient-centric view combined with the shift from care to prevention and wellness

We are on the verge of a new era in computing, in which innovative software applications on intelligent devices (clients), complemented by Internet-based data storage and services (the cloud), will offer individuals and organizations increased control over their information, and provide more intuitive and integrated services across computers, cell phones and other devices.

These advances will help individuals to become more productive and enable organizations of every size to become more agile, innovative, and collaborative. In healthcare, this next generation of computing holds enormous potential to open new frontiers, empowering individuals, healthcare organizations and governments to customize computing experiences to meet their specific needs.

The infusion of intelligence and connectivity into a wide range of devices, complemented by Internet-scale services, will create a new paradigm for computing based on the concept of "client plus cloud." This will allow governments to reduce IT costs while improving the patient (for which read consumer) experience, leading to better outcomes, more control, more convenience, better service, and ultimately better value for money.

We also see benefits for physicians as knowledge workers. As professionals they will be increasingly getting the right data in the right format at the right time, enabling them to provide the best treatment and preventive care.

eHealth is also about ensuring that every patient has a single holistic view of his/her medical history, covering all treatments and interventions, and not a paper trail spread across hospital departments and specialties, with vital records lost in the back of filing cabinets.

Beyond its ability to make existing systems far more efficient, eHealth applies ICT to improve access to healthcare for many more people while controlling costs and providing better quality of care.

Telemedicine, for example, enables patients to have a consultation with hospital-based specialists over a video link from their GP's surgery, permits X-rays and magnetic resonance images to be sent for analysis by specialists, and allows the results of diagnostic tests to be instantly transmitted. This means patients can monitor chronic conditions themselves at home.

Indeed, one of the most important developments arising from eHealth is the prospect of giving individuals the information and the tools they need to monitor their own health, and to support disease prevention programmes.

Whereas currently the providers are at the centre of the healthcare universe, and doctors and nurses are in control of the patient experience, individuals will be at the centre and empowered to take control of their own wellbeing.

eHealth is also about managing the information in ways that will increasingly allow our societies to focus on anticipation, prevention and wellness rather than on care and treatments once a disease is in train. eHealth systems will also pull together all the medical information that clinicians need to keep on top of the developments in their fields, backed up by decision-support search tools to enable them to apply this and move from being medical practitioners treating illness, to knowledge workers using information to maintain health.

Finally, at a systems level we see a learning healthcare system, which measures everything, identifies errors and makes improvements in order to deliver value within institutions and across institutional boundaries.

Building on this wave of innovation, the shift to a patient-centric healthcare system will be driven by software and services that increase efficiency, collaboration and decision-making among providers and promote involvement and lifestyle changes by individuals. Obviously, technology is not the only driver; there will be a long-term process that impacts personal attitudes, business models and public perceptions.

At Microsoft, we have a powerful vision for how technology can improve healthcare. This new system will enable a data-centred approach to healthcare that shifts the priorities from treatment and cure to prevention and lifelong wellness.

Why eHealth matters

It is hard to overestimate what is at stake here.

The need to reform healthcare is well known. Developed economies are already finding it hard to maintain standards of healthcare on existing budgets. Now payers are facing a huge dose of extra cost as, building on advances in biotechnology, pharmaceuticals, imaging, diagnostics and other fields, medical technology is delivering the potential for new treatments and diagnostics. eHealth stands out as a way to improve service and raise efficiency.

The problems are big. Europe should be celebrating the increasing lifespan of its citizens but instead is daunted by the cost of caring for an ageing population. By 2050, a third of the population will be over 60, an increase of 44 percent over 2006. The number over 80 years of age will increase by 180 percent. It is well known that the prevalence of most chronic conditions increases with age. Cancer and cardiovascular disease in the over-65s account for three-quarters of deaths across Europe. Demographic change is now combining with a recession that seems certain to threaten healthcare budgets, putting vulnerable groups at greater risk.

In the U.S. the problem is even starker. Healthcare spending there is growing at the fastest rate in history, and will reach $2.4 trillion this year. Its share of the country's gross domestic product is already four times that of defence. The bill is expected to grow to more than $4.3 trillion a year by 2017.

Martin Denz, President of the European Health Telematics Association (EHTEL), which represents interests from across the range of eHealth, argues that a major shift in perception is needed. Healthcare not only involves the practice of medicine; it is about how a healthy population generates a strong economy. The benefits of eHealth are two-fold: budgets are spent more productively, and eHealth can become an important export earner and a major source of new jobs and economic growth. Consider chronic diseases, which account for over 75% of healthcare spending. Even though most care for chronic diseases occurs at home, data from at-home care is not integrated with data available at the hospital or at the doctor's office. Individuals and providers would all benefit if, for example, patients with diabetes could upload their blood glucose readings to a Web site that offered personalized advice and guidance; receive information alerts regarding changes in recommended treatment or behaviour; share their results with a supportive community of fellow patients; and securely transmit readings to their clinician. Patients would have more information on how to manage their condition, would be in a better position to prevent acute incidents, and would need to make fewer trips to the doctor. Treating physicians would have a greater ability to understand their patients' health over time, allowing them to identify the best treatment for existing patients and to help people who are at risk of developing the disease in the future.

Some of the challenges of eHealth and the opportunity to overcome them

So, the health challenge is obvious. Then, there is the eHealth challenge.

Here is a basic paradox. Health is one of the most information-intensive sectors. But health services cannot manage and apply information in the ways the manufacturing and retail sectors have been doing for decades. This very backwardness means the health sector now has great potential to boost the efficiency and quality of its service. eHealth is one of the keys to unlock such potential.

However, as often happens at the early stages of any innovation, a succession of patchy strategies, botched implementations, cost overruns and dissatisfied users means that at best there is scepticism, and at worst a complete lack of understanding and even faith, in ICT-driven health reform among Europe's healthcare stakeholders. As a result, while the technology solutions are available, there is a vicious circle of technical and cultural obstacles that must be tackled before eHealth benefits can be realised in Europe.

Our current health system is built around the idea of a specific provider prescribing specific treatment for a specific condition. Patients' health data is locked inside each provider's silo, without being connected or shared. Physicians are forced either to make treatment and prescription decisions without all available clinical data, or else to waste time and resources attempting to aggregate data. MedStar Health's Washington Hospital Center estimates that 60% of a clinician's time is spent searching or waiting for information, with only 16% spent on direct patient care.

The right investments in eHealth can tear down these silos, offering patients and doctors a holistic picture of a patient's health history and thereby improving care.

Underlying all of this is a need to better connect health organizations and enable them to share data easily and efficiently. Having access to a patient's lifetime record of treatments, prescriptions and tests will enable individuals and their healthcare providers to make better medical decisions that improve outcomes and reduce wasteful spending.

This will require a new orientation—one that empowers consumers to be the stewards of their own health information and regards personal medical data as an asset to be managed over time and shared appropriately with those who support patients in making health decisions.

However, health services analysts point to cultural issues such as professional vested interests and the need to ensure patient confidentiality as an explanation for this lag. Data protection is paramount, of course, but there need to be incentives to share data and make it available at the appropriate time and place. This requires a focus on making systems interoperate and an insistence that vendors separate data from applications.

Another impediment to eHealth innovation is the traditional structure of many healthcare systems. Most care is delivered in the same context—of general practitioners' surgeries, accident and emergency, outpatients and hospital wards—as in the 19th century.

Then there is the view of patients themselves: too many think "risk" when they are presented with new technologies. This was identified as an invisible barrier by the European Commission in a report, "Future challenges for EU health and consumer policies."

Innovative solutions developed initially—and deployed successfully—in the U.S. and Canada, such as HealthVault, Microsoft's platform for consumer empowerment and engagement, with and through their personal health data, are leading the way in showing how to overcome the barrier of perceived risks. HealthVault, an Internet-based privacy and security-enhanced data storage and sharing platform, allows individuals to store copies of their health records from providers, plans, pharmacies, schools, government or employers; upload data from home health devices such as blood glucose monitors and digital scales; provide data to health care providers, coaches and trainers; and access information, products and services to help improve their health.

Microsoft's HealthVault was developed in cooperation with leading privacy advocates, security experts and dozens of the world's leading healthcare organisations to enhance privacy while providing individuals with control of their own health records.

Dr. Deborah Peel, founder of the Patient Privacy Rights Foundation, says Microsoft is the first major technology company to engage with the Coalition for Patient Privacy in a meaningful way. "The privacy protections built into HealthVault reflect the privacy principles of the Coalition. HealthVault prohibits onward transfer of data without explicit informed consent; its contractual obligations with advertisers require protection of any data transferred from the platform; its privacy policy is simple and easy to understand," she says.

"That means consumers finally have a trusted place to store their personal health information that will not be data-mined, because they alone control it. Microsoft's use of strong privacy principles including the principles of the

Coalition, its ongoing relationship with consumer advocates, and its commitment to independent third-party audits set a new standard for privacy protections in health information technology."

Some EU countries are already looking at this solution with great interest and exploring appropriate ways to tailor it and deploy it at national level, in cooperation with national stakeholders.

Along with consumers, hospitals have a crucial need to access, consolidate and share health data. In 2008 Microsoft launched Amalga, a data aggregation and health intelligence solution, in the U.S. Amalga aggregates and stores information from a hospital or health system's legacy systems, delivering a paradigm shift in how organizations can use the data housed in existing systems to drive change, discovery and innovation. Amalga allows agile use of information because it (1) captures all data in one place in real_time, including scans, images, device data and any other type of electronic data; (2) makes it easier to uncover relationships and advances discovery and diagnosis because it allows end_users to pose questions that either would not be apparent, or would not be answerable without the intervention of IT; and (3) provides a different approach to interfacing and integrating disparate data sources, reducing complexity and adding value.

Amalga and HealthVault are now being applied in areas such as ongoing chronic disease management, pre-registration, discharge management, data sharing with primary care providers, medication reconciliation and much more, to enable a seamless information exchange.

In 2009 Microsoft introduced Amalga Life Sciences, a new software system designed to transform healthcare and life science research data into the critical knowledge needed for the discovery of new personalized treatments. Microsoft Amalga Life Sciences 2009 helps organizations across the life sciences to advance to the next level of research capability by connecting data and investigators in new ways—through novel storage capabilities, ontology management functions and a semantic query environment powered by a next-generation reasoning engine.

To overcome barriers, we need policies that help support the new frontier of eHealth

As we move forward, we will expand our products and develop a new generation of software and services to help to support and speed the move towards efficient, data-driven medicine.

We recognize the need to support the technology-neutral policy goals and criteria that these systems should meet—such as those relating to security, privacy, interoperability and total cost of ownership. This can help to open the door to all companies to compete in the eHealth market and create the widest benefits for consumers. In specific terms we recommend:

♦ **Policies to ensure data can be moved seamlessly between different systems by requiring vendors to separate data from applications.** One of the key elements to overcoming technology barriers in data access, consolidation and sharing is to promote interoperability of eHealth systems, thus enabling information to move from one system to another. Interoperability also makes it possible to deal efficiently with public health emergencies and to improve evidence and knowledge creation in health research.

Microsoft is committed to the development of interoperability standards and works with the rest of the industry to reach consensus on such standards. But the requirement to be able to exchange healthcare data is urgent and a migration path is needed now. Today, data is too often used for a single application, or purpose, and then discarded. We can use metadata—the details that describe the data and how it was captured—to make patient information available for reuse, regardless of its original application or purpose. By requiring vendors to supply IT products that allow data transfer to and from other applications, we can get data moving between different systems before the emergence of standards that might take years to formulate.

Of course, the hurdles to interoperability in healthcare are higher than elsewhere. "First, you are dealing with personal data about medical conditions, so you only want to share it with authorised people," says Ilias Iakovidis, Deputy Head of Unit, ICT for Health at the European Commission. In other areas, such as finance, confidentiality is important too, but the information is not as complex. Numbers and simple concepts on one machine can, with appropriate security, be readily transmitted to another machine.

In healthcare, it is far more difficult to preserve the meaning and integrity of medical information when it goes from one system to another. A doctor's report in one electronic health record in one system is not easily understood and automatically translated by another doctor's system. The consequences of error could be grave—quite literally.

Interoperability is also key to building a pan-European market for eHealth. In Europe this is being realized thanks to the EU Commission's new "Lead Markets Initiative," which aims to use public procurement budgets, standardization and regulation to create market demand for innovative products and services in important industrial and social areas, including health.

With more than a dozen Member States working to set up electronic health records, the Commission is trying to ensure that these systems can work together. Its recommendations on cross-border interoperability of electronic health records, published in July 2008, aim to provide the basic principles and guidelines to enable doctors to access the records of patients, wherever the information may be located in Europe.

In support of this, the Commission is sponsoring the €22 million European Patient Smart Open Services (epSOS) project, of which Microsoft is a partner and strong supporter. epSOS is co-funded by the Commission and countries that have national electronic health records projects, along with the suppliers installing them, to demonstrate the benefits of interoperability. epSOS will work to ensure compatibility of electronic medical information, regardless of language or sophistication of technology, without having to establish a common system throughout Europe. This is the first time that the Commission has attempted to set out the steps needed to ensure compatibility between different national systems.

♦ Establishing and maintaining trust

For a connected health ecosystem to succeed, participants must be willing to share health data, and that willingness depends on whether they trust that their privacy will be protected. To establish and maintain this trust, software and services in the connected health ecosystem must offer *transparency*—to ensure that patients, physicians and providers understand how the data will be collected, who will have access to it and what it will be used for. They must also offer patients and providers *control* over the data—so patients can decide when and under what circumstances it will be shared, and providers can manage the data in a way that complies with applicable laws, regulations and policies. Effective *security* mechanisms are also needed to give stakeholders the confidence to embrace new software and service innovations without worrying about data breaches, identity theft and security flaws.

These principles—transparency, control and security—must be at the foundation of a system that supports today's complex mixture of legacy technical solutions and business models.

As a company that has long focused on using software to transform businesses and empower people, Microsoft believes that a combination of powerful software and rich Internet services—what we refer to as Software-plus-Services, has the potential to make the future we describe a reality by encouraging better outcomes and innovation, connecting patient data, and empowering consumers to be stewards of their own health.

♦ The need for a health-friendly user interface

For some, the biggest and most significant technical barrier to the deployment of eHealth systems on the frontline of healthcare, as opposed to the backroom management of information, is in data input and output. The keyboard and the mouse just aren't appropriate for healthcare. Voice input provides part of the answer, but digitising voice into free text does not provide structured data.

Microsoft is making a significant contribution here, collaborating with the UK's National Health Service on the development of the Common User Interface. This is the eHealth equivalent of the desktop in Microsoft Windows—enabling healthcare staff of many different technical competences, and with many different job functions, to use any computer, in any medical area.

♦ Shaping a single European market in healthcare

A central role for eHealth will be to support people in managing their own healthcare from home, within their own country but also across Europe.

The potential of this was highlighted in the last Euro Health Consumer Powerhouse ranking of Europe's national systems according to their attitudes to patients/consumers, published in November 2008. The analysis included measures of eHealth for the first time, and concluded that ICT is a key factor in the consumer-friendliness of healthcare systems, supporting partnership between the individual and the care system, and closing the gap between patients and professionals.

"Information will re-shape healthcare in the way we have seen in other major service industries," says Johan Hjertqvist, president of the Health Consumer Powerhouse, a leading provider of information and analysis of European healthcare.

Hjertqvist notes that at present it is essentially impossible to get any type of official data on the quality of cardiovascular healthcare in most European countries. Yet without such information there is little opportunity to increase the quality of that care. "After four years of comparison we now see the leading healthcare systems starting to adopt consumer trends. The leaders aim to support choice by providing information and, via consumer priorities, creating pressure for improvement of services and quality of care," says Hjertqvist.

"From this perspective it becomes evident that eHealth is a spearhead to radically reduce costs, open up the possibility of rapid access to treatment and improve patient safety."

The shift from patient care to individual wellness

Technology has long since transformed how we work, play and communicate. It is now poised to revolutionize our health for the better. Advances in genomics and diagnostics technology are making it possible to spot diseases earlier and treat them more effectively.

Machine learning and other techniques borrowed from computer science are helping scientists conduct more effective research and speed the development of drugs and other treatments. Patients are increasingly empowered by technologies that help them to cope with chronic conditions and maintain lifelong wellness—for example, glucose meters that help manage diabetes, and exercise equipment that monitors vital signs and keeps track of progress against personal fitness plans.

But a more remarkable transformation is yet to come. Advanced software and services that connect a wide range of medical technologies and data sources into a seamless whole will give patients, providers and payers a complete picture of health. This will support a patient-focused approach to medicine that shifts the priorities of healthcare from treatment and cure to prevention and lifelong wellness.

Whereas currently the providers are at the centre of the healthcare universe, and doctors and nurses are in control of the patient experience, individuals will be at the centre and empowered to take control of their own wellbeing.

At the same time, a rich marketplace of information, resources and services will increase efficiency and reduce costs across the spectrum of care. Clinicians will get the data and tools needed to provide the best treatment and will have the incentive to focus on preventive care. eHealth will underpin a learning healthcare system that measures everything, identifies errors and makes constant improvements.

How we get to the eHealth future

Individuals are now poised to take greater responsibility for their overall health and wellness. Technology can drive this transformation by:

♦ **Encouraging better outcomes and more innovation.** Under today's fee-for-service payment system, most physicians are not reimbursed for telephone or email consultations, let alone for more advanced uses of technology. In contrast, providers who compete on price and quality are constantly looking for ways to improve service and to bundle procedures with services leveraging technology and communications.

♦ **Connecting patient data.** Because patients' health data is locked in silos, physicians are forced either to make treatment decisions based on incomplete data or else to waste time and resources aggregating information. A complete health history would enable providers to make better medical decisions, decrease wasteful spending and increase the quality of care.

♦ **Empowering consumers.** If consumers could connect all their health and wellness data electronically, share their data securely with different providers and keep it in one place over time, they would have information at their fingertips to make better choices about physicians, care options, and ways to improve their overall wellbeing.

THAIMA SAMMAN is Associate General Counsel at Microsoft in charge of driving Government Affairs and CSR activities across the European Union. Thaima Samman became a licensed attorney in 1996 with a specialized postgraduate diploma (DESS) in banking and financial law, as well as an advanced postgraduate diploma (DEA) in criminal policy and law in Europe, but she began her career as a founding member of a prominent French NGO, SOS Racism, having for its main goal to fight all forms of discrimination, devoting several years to its development before serving as a member of staff for Claude Bartolone, MP and former member of the French Government.

She practiced law at private firms, created a start-up and then joined Philip Morris as head of the Communications, Public and Regulatory Affairs Department at the French level. In 2003, she joined Microsoft France as the head of its legal and public affairs department, and then moved to Microsoft Europe, Middle East and Africa where she currently leads the Corporate Affairs Department in the region, driving and coordinating policy and CSR activities, in particular at the EU level. Thaima is also the founder of Women and Leadership in the Information Society (WIL) network working at the European level with high-level women from various industries, administration and NGO and has authored various publications on issues such as immigration and foreigners' rights, privacy issues, and information technology, recently publishing an article about young women in ICT. Thaima has been named a chevalier of the Ordre Nationale du Merite for the Republic of France.

ELENA BONFIGLIOLI is Director of Corporate Responsibility for Microsoft Europe, Middle East and Africa. Elena leads strategy, program development, partnership building and policy advocacy on Health, Education, Skills and Employability, Entrepreneurship and Accessibility. Elena has been with Microsoft for over six years in the role of Director CSR. She currently chairs various groups and advocacy organizations in the CSR and ICT areas. Elena was one of the founders of the European Alliance on Skills for Employability and she currently acts as Chair person. She also leads the Digital Europe i2010 Lisbon policy group. Elena also co-chairs the e-Skills Industry Leadership Board (ILB), a coalition of leading companies and stakeholders committed to developing e-skills for an inclusive and competitive Europe. Before joining Microsoft, Elena worked for the European Network on Corporate Responsibility (CSR Europe) as Programmes Director. Elena was one of the pioneers and founders of the European Academy of Business in Society and initially served EABiS as interim Director for the first year and a half of activity. Elena started her career working as a researcher for the Italian government and the University of Bologna in the field of fiscal economic reform. Elena holds a cum Laude degree in economics from the University of Modena, Italy, and a Master's degree in European studies from the College of Europe, in Belgium.

Chapter 12

From Clouds to Transparency in the Relationships Between Patient 2.0 & Health Care Practitioners

Philippe Scheimann, MSc MBA

Daniel Laury, M.D.

Introduction

This paper studies the nature of the relationship between patient 2.0 and health care practitioners with an emphasis on pharmacists and medical doctors located in France and in the U.S.

Background description

U.S. and French regulations regarding the healthcare market and the Web are rather different. U.S. doctors and pharmacist are allowed to advertise their services online and offline. There is strict regulation in France as well as cultural discomfort. U.S. and Canadian pharmacies are allowed to sell online drugs with prescriptions in contrast to Europe in toto.

A common theme in the U.S. and Europe deals with the lack of transparency regarding the prices of health services. As far as we know, there are virtually no websites that list the prices of consultations and medical procedures (treatments, services, operations…) whether it be in the U.S. or in Europe. With much efforts, it is possible to loop up the website (ameli.fr) of the French Social Security and see the prices of consultations by specialists and various technical acts. The information provided is still at its infancy.

Relationships between patient/healthcare practitioner

This chapter explores the nature of the relationships between patient and pharmacist on one hand, and between patient and medical doctor on the other.

Then, patient-to-patient relationships will be analyzed.

Based upon the transaction cost theory (7) and work by the late Professor

Ciborra (1), there is a need to study the level of uncertainty or complexity of the relationship as well as the behavioral uncertainty, level of trust and goal congruence between the parties.

Trends:

♦ Financial crisis: health budget limited

♦ Health Insurances: less reimbursement

♦ Growing use of the Net

♦ Privacy required regarding health personnal situation vs. use of Web 2.0 features

Some definitions related to health, the Web and transaction cost theory (alphabetical order)

Community

Group of people sharing the same interest. Howard Rheingold is supposedly the first to have introduced the notion of Virtual Community. Successful online communities are usually based upon real identities of the users and clear guidelines. There is the notion of a virtual medical community mostly for use of healthcare practitioners based on the same interest to improve the management of specific disease states.

Complexity

When dealing with complexity, we are talking about various levels of uncertainty. It is useful to differentiate between natural complexity and behavioral complexity. There is a need to study on one hand the complexity of the task and on the other hand the relationships between both parties that is the level of trust and goal congruence.

e-Identity: online and offline identity

Keeping an online Identity or e-Identity is not an easy challenge in most cases and it is even more difficult when dealing with health data, the identity of the patient and health care practitioners. Stealing identities and building online profiles of patients for business purposes are some of the common threats.

Health 2.0

Combination of health data and health information with (patient) experience through the use of ICT. It enables the individual to become an active and responsible partner in his/her own health and care pathway.

ICT

Information and Communication Technology

Internet-Web 2.0

Digital Age's philosopher (3) wrote: "This is the information age, we are knowledge workers, the Internet is a well of information, a knowledge fountain." The power of the Web to harness collective intelligence: users add value, innovation in assembly.

Patient 2.0

This expression brings together the status of a patient with Web 2.0 features. Patient 2.0 is no longer passive, but thanks to the Web 2.0, there is not only access to relevant and adequate information but also a possible active online involvement of the patient.

Privacy

Keeping a high level of privacy while being active on the Web is a challenge. It is all the more difficult when dealing with personal health information. People have the right not to reveal their health specifics and to maintain their privacy, but it is a complex process when being active online searching for specific information, asking questions, etc. The privacy issue starts, for example, when using Google while searching for specific topics. It continues with being active in a virtual community or social network.

Transaction

The authors are using the notion of transaction from the transaction cost theory (7). Similar to business arenas, any relationship between patient and health care practitioner can be defined as a set of transactions with relative level of uncertainty. A relationship between a patient and a healthcare professional is never neutral and is by nature hierarchal.

Trust

As we will see, trust is key when dealing with patient health care practitioners. Factors such as honesty, competency and fidelity need to be taken into consideration. (6) There are many articles that emphasize the importance of this "soft" criterion, which is usually difficult to deal with. See uncertainty goal congruence and level of trust.

User Generated Content (UGC)

UGC websites allow users to add content on their own so that it is possible to generate and gather in one place information that would not be accessible otherwise. For example, www.ComparSante.fr provides tools for users to enter the various prices for the same drugs sold in French pharmacies.

Uncertainty

The natural uncertainty and the behavioral uncertainty are the main factors affecting the

transaction between various parties. Uncertainty can be expressed in terms of complexity of the transaction and level of trust between the parties.

Transaction Costs

Transaction costs appear at each step of the relationship between patients and health care professionals. This ranges from finding the right practitioner, to contract, maintenance and closure of the relationship. There are different costs related to each phase of the transaction:

> **Search and information costs**—These are costs related to determining that the required goods are available on the market, finding a practitioner, checking the credentials, finding the pharmacist who has the most attractive price for a specific drug, etc. Information Technology and the Web can play a major role for reducing those costs. For instance, it is not rare that potential patient check the Web for credentials (Googling the name of the practitioner) and start an email correspondence asking for various details before deciding to come to the consultation.

> **Bargaining costs**—These are the costs related to set up an appropriate contract. Due to the use of insurances, certain costs are less relevant in the patient/healthcare professional relationship. However, it does happen with the costs of technical procedures and consultations of specialists mostly on a one on one basis.

> **Policing and enforcement costs**—The costs of making sure the other party complies with the terms of the contract, and taking appropriate action (possibly legal action) if this turns out not to be the case.

Use of Information Technology in the transaction costs

Effective use of IT can reduce various costs such as finding, contacting and even meeting a practitioner. Note that an in-depth review of telemedicine is beyond the scope of this chapter.

Analysis of each position in the case of the relationships with the medical doctor and pharmacist

Trust from a health care provider's perspective is an important component of

Table 1. *Relationships: patient/healthcare professional.*

care. Establishing trust has benefits to the provider, the patient and society in general. Medical ethics deals with decision making outside of strictly practicing care. There has been a shift towards Principle-Based Ethics in which four principles are promulgated:

1. Patient *autonomy* involves a person's right to guide their own care. A person has the capability and, indeed, the right to educate themselves about their situation, choose from options and ultimately decide on a course of action. Often, they turn to the internet to find this information.

2. *Beneficience* is when a provider must consider and act in the patient's best interest.

3. *Nonmaleficence* consists of the principle of causing no harm. A provider is expected to minimize injury and pain to their patient.

4. The fourth component is *justice*. Here, care must be considered within the confines of our society; thinking about limited resources, triage issues, society's morals, etc.

Trust comes into play in the last three principles. By establishing a trusting relationship, the patient will accept that the provider is considering their best interests (beneficience), will not cause them undue harm (nonmaleficence) and has weighed in on the best option for them (justice).

Besides the moral issues involved, there are some very practical outcomes that come within a trust relationship.

From a patient's perspective, we can see that they will have less anxiety about the course of care. If a trusted provider recommends a hysterectomy, for example, rather than a trial of a hormone therapy, the patient will feel comfortable that the decision was not unduly influenced by the financial reimbursement expected. If the practitioner advises a woman to divorce a spouse, there is the expectation that her best interests are at heart and that the psychiatrist's personal issues are not influencing the recommendation.

Patients are also more likely to follow through with a medical plan when there is trust. Physicians are taught that up to 50% of prescriptions are not even filled by patients after an encounter. Non-compliance is a real problem in healthcare, especially with chronic disease treatments. Where there is trust, there can be better outcomes.

Healthcare providers can also expect advantages. Certainly, advising a patient to follow through with a plan is much easier if the trust is already established. There is less need to convince or cajole a patient that it is in their best interest to follow through with the recommendation. This helps in terms of provider satisfaction, favorable outcomes and clinic efficiency.

Legally, patients are less likely to litigate where there is a trusting relationship. As defensive medicine is a worldwide problem, this may help reduce unnecessary ordering of potentially painful and time consuming tests. It can save time for staff in performing tests as well as for providers needing to overdocument patient notes. Less legal costs will help the tort system function better and improve insurance efficiency.

What can a provider do to establish trust? What can a patient do to find a trustworthy pharmacist? What metrics are available to search out an honorable physician? How does a medical office maintain trust?

Prospective patients generally rely on personal references. Indeed, in my medical practice, approximately 80% of new patient visits come from word of mouth; someone recommended us to that person. By being trustworthy to a current patient, it is likely that they will speak highly of us to a future patient. When a patient's personal physician sets up an appointment with another physician, this implies that they have trust in that specialist. Similarly, if a doctor sends a client to a specific pharmacy for a prescription, it is understood that there is a trusting relationship there. Interactive websites offer an alternative way of getting personal references to help find a trusted practitioner.

Trust can also be established by credentials. The granting body, in effect, is stating that this provider can be trusted based on certain criteria. These may involve diplomas, awards, membership in medical boards and societies, magazine and journal editors' acceptance of manuscripts, inclusion in various groups... In this information age, prospective patients often look online for the provider's website, online journals, interviews and webTV. It is understood, however, that there is misleading information also promulgated online. Rave reviews may not be accurate, and complaints may be related to poor outcomes rather than poor medical care. Most readers intuitively appreciate the fact that every unhappy client will complain to nine people while satisfied people only tell four. In a domain where there is tremendous lack of oversight, it is often up to the provider to respond or even correct misleading information.

A classic medical scenario is when an independent company rates physicians based on complications. Though Doctor **A** may have a higher number of complications than Doctor **B**, it would be important to note that Doctor **A** may also see many more patients than Doctor **B** or that they take care of more complicated cases. Physicians may also be limited in their ability to respond to every complaint as they may not have the time to mine the web. Sometimes, there is no way to respond to the information as the site is set up strictly as a sounding board for patients.

The third most common was to establish trust comes from the patient's personal evaluation. It is often said that the physician's staff sets the stage for the patient. A courteous and caring front office person will help establish a positive relationship even before meeting the provider. The office location and décor can likewise set up expectations. A tasteful office in a good location suggests that the practitioner is doing well and, therefore, is likely to have had good relationships with patients in the past. The provider's demeanor is critical to establishing trust. Is there eye contact with the patient? Are they dressed appropriately? Do they look tired? Is the provider obese or unhealthy appearing? Are they looking at their watch often? What do they say about other providers' care? Many physicians offer a complimentary "meet and greet" appointment to make sure that there is a good fit. I commonly see new clients who have already "interviewed" me via email and/or videoconferencing. Tours of a potential pharmacy can be conducted in person or by virtual reality.

There is a fine line between advertisement, self-promotion and education. In France, for example, physicians are not legally able to advertise, whereas in the U.S., it is common. For example, approximately 10% of a plastic surgeon's income is spent in promotion. One of the authors (DL) has a television program which is educational, however, clearly it helps the practice grow.

In addition, federal rules in the U.S. prohibit health care entities from releasing a patient's protected information inappropriately. It is, therefore, difficult to advertise a client's excellent response to a provider's care.

Another limitation deals with physician charging structure. Generally, providers have limited discussing fees in an open forum. Fears include allegations of price fixing or overcharging and undercharging the competition. There has been a great deal of debate over the idea of offering a money back guarantee. While all of the above is standard practice for other types of businesses, medical care operates under a different set of rules. This can make it difficult for consumers to find out information that may help them make an educated decision.

Back to trust parameters. There are some that a provider cannot change. Certain patients may be more comfortable with one gender over another. The provider's perceived age can influence a patient's trust. Religious affiliation and sexual orientation can likewise impact on trust. Sometimes trust is not with a provider per se, but rather with the company or group. Look at online pharmacies. Here, the relationship is between the patient and the corporation; there may be no actual pharmacist to discuss things with. The trust involves the expectation that the prescription is filled accurately with a quality product at a reasonable price.

Relationships: Patient/MD specialist

Table 2. *Relationships: Patient/MD specialist.*

Hi	Not so Stable 'Cloudy'	Clear but costs to reach & maintain this situation
Trust level	Patient may switch doctors Use of minute clinics in malls	Key Problem 'Very Cloudy' "Patients with a lower level of trust in their physician are more likely to report that requested or needed services are not provided".?
Lo	**Lo**	**Hi**

Task complexity/uncertainty

Limitations of trust

There are times, however, that trust is not a priority and, thus, search and information costs are not relevant. Take, for example, the case when someone is in a car accident and is cared for by emergency providers. There is no time for checking on credentials or consideration of personal preferences.

Low complexity of the treatment

When a treatment is standard or of a low complexity, trust parameter may not be relevant, and the cost may become a major factor for decision making. Patients may accept a provider who instills less trust in them. As an example, witness the birth of the clinics in the U.S. found in shopping malls or department stores where diagnosis and treatment is available on the spot.

Growing complexity of the treatment

As the complexity of the situation increases, trust issues may become more important. The practitioner must evaluate all available information as it is critical to the proper management of the case. Trust issues come into play when the provider presents a medical management plan to the patient. The rapport will improve compliance and, therefore, the outcome. Without the trust, a patient may end up jeopardizing their health by not following through with the medical advisements (6).

Relationships Patient—Pharmaceuticals

Pharmaceuticals are under a great deal of scrutiny lately given that there are so many opportunities for mistakes. In the U.S. and Canada, prescriptions may be obtained online. We often read about someone dying from an

Table 3. *Relationships: Patient/Pharmacist.*

Hi		
	Allows pharmacist to advise, suggest another drug: e.g. generic substitute	Steady relationship
Trust level	Patient/consumer could decide where to buy if only there was market transparency	Potential problems with pharmacist: price bargaining, service etc.
Lo		
	Lo	Hi

Complexity/uncertainty

overdosage, impurity, interaction or even the wrong prescription being filled. Drugs can be a low risk or high risk situation depending on the product. A simple antibiotic for acne generally can be considered low risk because the failure of treatment may be benign. However, if someone has a true drug allergy and receives the wrong drug, this can cause fatal anaphylaxis. Patients have been able to obtain medications from some online pharmacies even without prescriptions. Due to the necessity of regulation, various groups are getting into the field of patient advocacy and education, including pharmacy checker, IPABC, CIPARx and others. Due to the lack of transparency in the pricing of drugs and medical acts in pharmacies, various groups are entering this domain.

Switching positions (from unstable to stable)

1. High complexity → Low complexity

In situations where trust levels cannot be ameliorated, there is the possibility of decreasing the complexity. In medical care, one option is to parse the problem into its constituent subsets. An example might be where a patient is on a ventilator after a stroke. We may have a neurologist come in to consult on the brain function, a physical therapist to help with keeping the joints flexible, a nutritionist to manage intravenous feeding, a pulmonologist to deal with the lung function, a pharmacist to manage all of the medications, etc. Another example would be when a patient receives multiple medications from multiple providers. Not only can there be redundancy but also serious interactions. A pharmacist could interact with the practitioners to improve patient compliance (once a day drug vs. three times a day), increase safety (suggest a less toxic alternative) and decrease poor combinations (alerting the provider of possible catastrophic consequences).

2. Low level of trust → High level of trust using Information Technology

Apart from the human and psychological aspects of raising trust from the point of view of a practitioner, an intelligent use of the technology can help raise the trust for the patient. Health practitioners can use ITC (e.g. Internet TV for broadcasting programs, CRM tools and more) in order to reach a high level of trust with the patients and help them deal with the uncertainty of the situation the best way as possible.

Relationship patient 2.0/patient2.0

Use of the Web

Patients can use the Web in order to improve their health situation. They may have a high or a low trust level relationship with a health care practitioner involving a complex or simple transaction. A recommendation is to use the potential of Web 2.0 and the interest of the whole in order to gather "hidden" information, such as the range of prices of drugs, medical acts and

Table 4. *Relationships: Patient 2.0/Patient 2.0.*

Hi	Stable area	Word of mouth from family/friends ('real life community') with exceptions from social networks with very clear guidelines. There is the danger of getting mislead.
Lo	Social networks including anonymous inputs can be useful for asking questions related to hard facts such as prices of drugs, consultations, and medical acts.	Dangerous area where people will not be telling the truth etc. Hearsay from the web rumors...

(Trust level)

Lo ———————————— **Hi**

Task complexity/uncertainty

consultations of specialists. However, this potential does not cover the field of information about the practitioners (reputation, quality of service, professionalism, etc.)

Regarding the framework of task complexity vs. level of trust, a careful use of ITC will allow a reduction in transaction costs, thus forming more successful relationships. Clients and health care practitioners can then avoid pitfalls and strengthen their positions.

In the matrix above, we can see that in a low complexity situation, such as picking a less expensive pharmacy, the trust issues are of minimum importance. If one web posting deviates significantly from the majority of the others, this will not lead a patient astray. It only gets to be problematic when the complexity increases or the trust issue importance increases.

As an example, let's say that a patient posts a statement to the effect that a given medication gave them a serious side effect (e.g. Nitrofurantoin and lung damage). Another patient with a complicated health problem that requires that pharmaceutical may read and accept unconditionally the post and refuse treatment. This may lead to dire consequences. Commonly, we also find that a "friend" or a "family member" describes horrendous outcomes from therapies which understandably scare off patients from legitimate treatments. The ability to be anonymous on the Web also reduces the trust issues.

From a high trust perspective, when the posting individual has been identified as a trusted source, such as an author or professional, their input can actually be more damaging if it goes against the legitimate advice of a treating provider. Often, the commenting individual has no access to the patient's medical record and has not met and examined them. This may lead to inappropriate comments.

Conclusion

Web 2.0 and privacy in the healthcare arena do not live well together. There is still a need to create innovative social health related communities empowering the patients and healthcare practitioners while keeping trust and privacy respected. In the meantime, it is at least possible to provide a mechanism for patients to improve the transparency regarding health care prices.

PHILIPPE SCHEIMANN, MSc MBA, Founder of ComparSante, a French start-up developing a user generated content website providing price comparisons of health related products. He is also Chief Technologist at POLITECH Institute & CEO of Ayala Alternative Organizational Consulting. He is a Management Technologist, Internet Veteran and Social Entrepreneur. He has vast experience in management consulting, in creating and launching virtual communities for collaboration and conflict resolution for international projects with NGOs as well as in the business sector.

DANIEL LAURY, M.D., a pioneer in women's health, is a board-certified Gynecologist. He graduated from Albert Einstein College of Medicine in 1988. After completing his internship and residency in Pennsylvania, he came to Medford, Oregon. In addition to running his busy private practice, he also hosts a medical educational TV program, has been involved in many research protocols and enjoys writing. He has just published the book *Senior Sex, Answers to your questions from a geriatric gynecologist.*

REFERENCES

Ciborra, Claudio U. Teams, market and systems University Press, Cambridge U.K 1993

Lodewijk Bos, 2008. Patient 2.0 Empowerment, SWWS08 Proceedings

Gerry McGovern, March 03, 1997 New Thinking: The Internet: sofa or stage?

Chapter 13

Taiwan's National Health Informatics Project, 2008–2011

Charng-Er Shyu, Counselor and Director, Health Informatics Center in the Department of Health, Taiwan

Background

The Department of Health (DOH) of Taiwan's Executive Yuan conducted the Current Status Survey of Computerization of Medical Records by Medical Institutions in December 2005.[1] The survey referenced the five stage definitions of EMR development from the US Medical Record Association. As shown in Figure 1, approximately 95.4% of the hospital EMR development in Taiwan is still in Stage 1 to Stage 3; 43.7% of the clinics have not computerized medical records and 55.6% of the clinics are still in Stage 2. Stage 2 indicates hospital

Figure 1. *Result of Current Status Survey of Computerization of Medical Records by Medical Institutions in Taiwan 2005.*

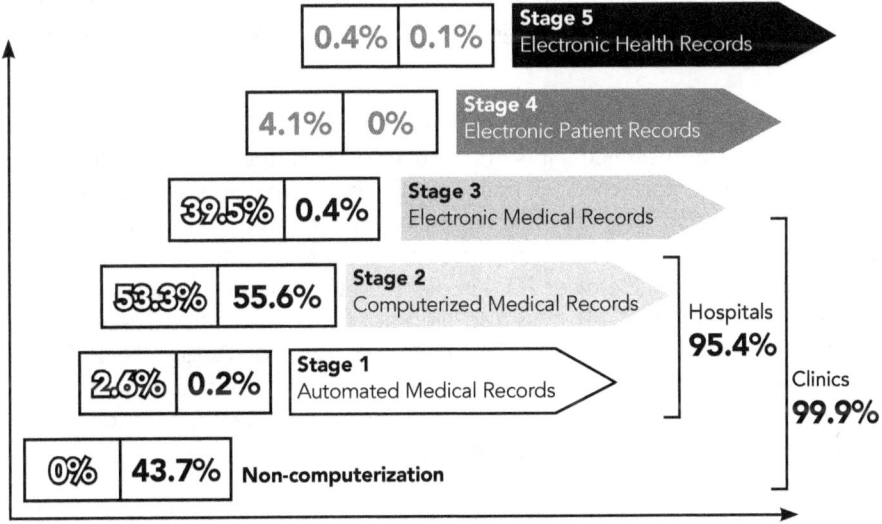

Respondents: 460 hospitals and 4,032 clinics

data requires further integration, while Stage 3 indicates hospitals have already established a platform for patients' integrated medical records but not yet available with sharing of medical record information with other hospitals via the internet. Thus, there is still room for computerization of medical records for the current 500 and more hospitals and over 19,000 clinics.

Regarding laws and regulations governing electronic medical records, presently there is the Regulation of EMR Production and Management by Medical Institutions, which stipulates that hospitals should comply with the regulation of information security and electronic signature while adopting EMR. However, laws and regulations pertaining to public health and medical care privacy protection and information security are scattered in the Computer-Processed Personal Data Protection Act, Medical Care Act, Physicians Act, Nursing Personnel Act and Civil Law, etc. It still requires review of their adequacy so that the public's EMR can be protected by laws and regulations.

Regarding public health service, the DOH started promotion of providing the public with internet services by public health bureaus in 2003, and established a host of information systems with different functions in 2004 and 2005 to truly improve the efficiency of claims and applications. However, a review of today's public health information internet services shows that the scope and service items are beyond the anticipated scope and complexities. As regards the national health indicator design and applications, health data collection is mostly respectively carried out by the Centers of Disease Control (CDC), the Bureau of Health Promotion (BHP), the DOH Statistics Office and the Bureau of National Health Insurance (NHI). This often caused duplication in collection of similar information or production of similar health indices, which are not only time and manpower consuming, the national health information scattered in various units also restricts the collection of health indices and value-added applications of future innovations.

Therefore, to provide continuous medical care for patients and more convenient public health services, it is imperative to boost the infrastructure for promotion of EMR enforcement of hospitals. Furthermore, we need an integration mechanism to plan for the public health information system and the health repository to guarantee privacy of personal health information. To this end, the DOH commenced in October 2004 in planning the National Health Information Project (NHIP) (2008-2011), and also filed application with the Executive Yuan for the project in 2005 and 2006, which was approved on August 14, 2007. The government will play the role of enabler in the creation of a national health information development environment and important infrastructure for the utilization of health and medical information.

1. NHIP Objectives

The primary objectives of NHIP are to create a national health information development environment, promote important infrastructure of health and medical care information, foster use of the information technology by Taiwan's health and medical circles, enhance the effective use of medical resources, medical care service quality and patient safety, and achieve the goal of building an interoperable lifelong e-health information infrastructure, under the prerequisite of guaranteeing personal privacy of the public.

2. NHIP Strategy and Budget

NHIP has formulated five major strategies to address the domestic EMR, medical and health information development issues to be respectively executed in five sub-projects. Annual budget requirement for the various sub-projects (as shown in Table 1) will ensure execution of the various tasks. The strategies are described below:

- ◆ The first strategy is to promote the adoption of EMR mainly through incentives of the policy side and administrative side and improvement of necessary infrastructure of EMR, and urge hospitals to accelerate EMR adoption in order to improve medical care quality and patient safety.

- ◆ The second strategy is promotion of a basic legal system for national health information primarily through review of ethical, legal and social issues (ELSI) related to NHIP and possible ELSI concern for various applications. Improvement of the required legal system entails privacy protection and a mechanism for regulating and reviewing information management in formulation and promotion of health information applications so as to achieve the purpose of guaranteeing health information security and privacy for the public.

- ◆ The third strategy is the establishment and operation of the Healthcare Certification Authority (HCA[2]). This is done primarily through provision of certification service for electronic medical documents, electronic signature and data encryption to ensure confidentiality of electronic medical information, integrity, signer's identity identification and non-repudiation.

- ◆ The fourth strategy is the deployment of public health information application service system. This is done primarily through review of current public health information service, flow and technology, under the prerequisite of guaranteeing personal privacy and permission of laws and decrees. Moreover, we need to build and improve the public health information correlation and exchange mechanism and the integrated application service architecture pertaining to medical and healthcare. This will provide public health information integrated services for the health authorities and medical institutions to satisfy requirements for real-time acquisition of public health information, and for analysis and decision-making support.

♦ The fifth strategy is promotion of value-added applications for health information with the purpose of improving integration of health information and innovation of value-added applications. The integrated information comprises of public health, medical and health care, social, economic and geographical information; and value-added application service comprises of public health decision-making, relevant academic research, medical and health care services and research and development and innovation of relevant industries.

Table 1. *NHIP Budget Summary Chart*

Unit: NT$ (thousand)

Sub-Project Name	2008	2009	2010	2011	Total
1. Promotion of the Adoption of EMR	158,480	43,708	35,000	50,000	287,188
2. Establishing the Basic Laws and Regulations for National Health Information Exchange	50	500	500	500	1,550
3. The Establishment and Operation of Healthcare Certification Authority	108,740	83,302	65,000	55,000	312,042
4. Deployment of Public Health Information Application Service System.	91,684	97,206	77,000	77,000	342,890
5. Promotion of Value-added Applications for health information	7,851	23,718	23,000	22,000	76,569
Total	**366,805**	**248,434**	**200,500**	**204,500**	**1,020,239**

3. NHIP Current Status and Development

The current status and development of the five NHIP sub-projects are described in the following:

3.1 Sub-project 1: Promotion of the Adoption of EMR

This sub-project can mainly be promoted in four dimensions, namely, legal side, security side, standards side and promotion side for EMR practice and applications. They are briefly described below:

Legal side: Mainly executed by sub-project 2. For details refer to section 4.2.

Security side: Improve the protective capability of hospital in EMR information security through a series of information security improvement projects. The primary tasks in 2009 are: (1) Scheduled to complete training of 400 hospital information security personnel to acquire certificates of leading auditor for ISO 27001⊠2005. The leading auditors will assist hospitals with building and promoting the information security management system. (2) Sponsor 80 seminars on hospital information security in order to elevate the consciousness and capability of hospital personnel for protection of medical care information and EMR security. (3) Provide accreditation service for information security management systems of 46 hospitals and encourage hospitals to setup their information security management system and get certification with the aim of building a safe and reliable information working environment. Aforementioned tasks will be continuously implemented in the coming years in view of practical need.

Standards side: Representatives of relevant associations and medical societies were invited to jointly amend and formulate 108 forms of EMR standard format in 2008 and 2009 according to medical care practice and application requirements. These forms will be converted into machine-readable formats. Also, we need to build a standard maintenance mechanism comprising of six steps, namely, proposal, draft, announcement, review, voting and promulgation. Moreover, we have to develop a standard EMR management system with registration and inquiry functions so as to ensure a consistent standard version of EMR and provide for inquiry by various circles. Hereafter, we will continue to amend in accordance with practical requirements so as to improve the domestic standard EMR format.

Promotion side: Since hospitals in Taiwan continue to use paper medical record examination for health insurance claim applications and hospital accreditation operation, the willingness for adoption of EMR by medical institutions is low. Therefore, it is necessary to improve relevant ancillary measures to enhance the practical effect of EMR adoption. Presently, the ongoing work is to provide hospitals accreditation standard and recommendations for the amendment of EMR quality scoring description. Also, we have to provide relevant technology and counseling for medium and small hospitals, which lack practical resources and technology for EMR implementation.

4.2 Sub-project 2: Establishing the Basic Laws and Regulations for National Health Information Exchange

This sub-project is primarily based on the practical requirements of hospitals to continuously amend the Regulation of EMR Production and Management for Medical Institutions. The focus of amendment is for maintenance and operation of EMR information security, adding of electronic signature and time-stamping with the purpose of ensuring public EMR information security and avoiding difference between the legal system and practice, which affect the original intention of legislation. Therefore, amendments were carried out twice respectively on December 25, 2008 and August 11, 2009. Hereafter, appropriate amendments will be carried out again in view of the circumstances of EMR implementation by the medical institutions.

4.3 Sub-project 3: The Establishment and Operation of Healthcare Certification Authority

In the initial period of promotion of EMR and NHI IC card, there was no Government Public Key Infrastructure (GPKI) certification mechanism, the DOH planned the Healthcare Certification Authority (HCA) by utilizing the Public Key Infrastructure (PKI) in 2002 in order to improve medical care information security and boost computerized applications of medical care information. To issue certificates for medical personnel and medical institutions, the HCA was officially commissioned on June 13, 2003 and issued the first generation healthcare certification IC card on August 22 of the same year. The HCA was officially put under the Government Root Certification Authority (GRCA) on August 19, 2008 and started to issue second generation healthcare certification IC cards.

As of July 31, 2009, a total of 157,992 first generation healthcare certification IC cards had been issued (including 142,576 medical personnel cards and 15,416 medical institution cards), and also a total of 61,925 second generation cards (including 54,443 medical personnel cards and 7,482 medical institution cards.) However, currently there are a total of 250,359 medical personnel in Taiwan with 117,404 of them who have never applied for healthcare certification IC cards. Henceforth, various propaganda and promotion activities will be planned for popularity of healthcare certification in order to accelerate the computerization of medical care service. Operation of HCA and issuance of healthcare certification IC cards will continue in 2010. However, the length of the user certification key will be adjusted from 1024 bits to 2048 bits and also simultaneously add and amend relevant encryption and decryption and signature programs.

4.4 Sub-project 4: Deployment of Public Health Information Application Service System

This sub-project is mainly for integrating the 50 information systems developed by the DOH and provided for use by the health authorities or by hospitals. The integrated information system will be gradually expanded and integrated into the public health information systems of the health authorities and promoted into single sign-on integration work. Furthermore, to avoid affecting operation of the current systems, particular consideration has been given to the architecture to meet requirements of openness, expandability, backup and balanced loading while planning for the public health information application service architecture.

Aside from completing more than 50% of integration of the public health information systems of affiliated organs of the DOH and the application service architecture of this project and the portals, partial replacement of the expired and unusable equipment and the equipment expansion installation work of this project will also be completed. In the coming years, we will continue to integrate the relevant public health information systems and improve the community medical healthcare institutions in using this project's integrated application service information. To satisfy the requirement of the public health authorities for public health information integrated services and real-time and correct acquisition of information, we have to elevate public health information analysis, evaluation and decision-making support, thereby providing the public the best healthcare service.

For gradual expansion of the project system construction, a project office was set up in 2008 and 2009 to review the current health indices and fundamental database content, improve data security and data quality, and collect requirements for health indices and fundamental databases from the various units of the DOH and the affiliated organs. In addition, the project office will plan for collective health indices, fundamental databases, setup of value-added application platform and coordination center, and carry out planning for risk evaluation and internal and external control mechanism.

Fundamental databases will be collected by the various units for the statistics office of the DOH for distributed architecture storage after encryption. If required in the future, the data will be linked after encryption in accordance with different application purposes. Depending on the requirement of value-added individual cases, the required data will be retrieved from the fundamental database for processing by the value-added application platform, including depersonalization, statistical analysis and fuzzification. Only then collective secondary data or statistical quantity will be stored into the health repository or for external provision after review. Index requirement, data processing steps, platform use and the content and method for external provision of statistical results must go through the health data value-added application committee and the advisory group, and review, supervision and control procedures of the working group and the coordination center. Its system architecture is shown in Figure 2 (see next page).

NHIP Expected Results

To accomplish the various sub-project objectives in an orderly and gradual manner and accomplish the final NHIP goal, NHIP has drafted yearly performance

Figure 2. *Value-added Application Architecture for NHIP Health Promotion.*

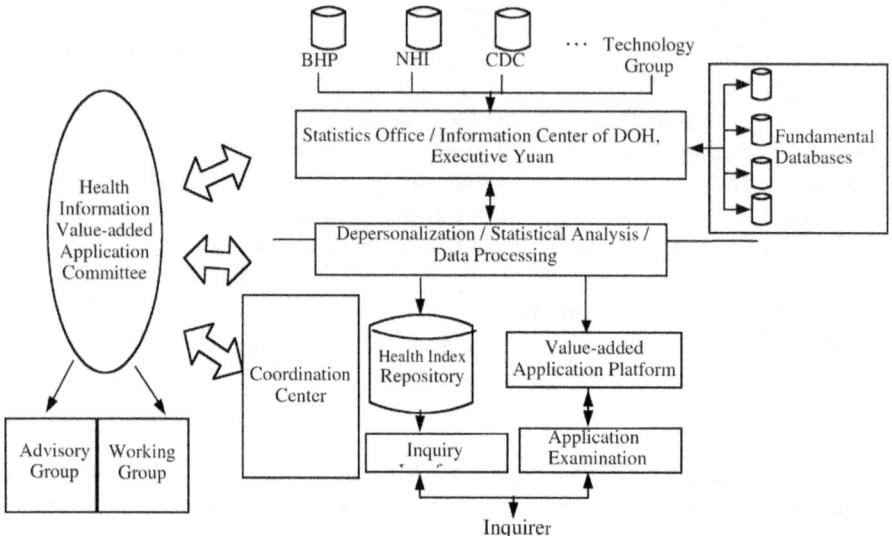

index objectives for 2008 to 2011. This is aimed to complete promotion of EMR adoption in 10% of the hospitals and 3% of the clinics in Taiwan and formulate of relevant laws and regulations and standards. In addition, promotion of second generation healthcare certification IC cards will accumulate to 100,000 cards, and achieve at least 90% in developing the function ratio of public health information integrated services and applied all health indices as defined by the World Health Organization (WHO) and the Organization for Economic Co-operation and Development (OECD).

Moreover, execution of this project will also bring following anticipated benefits:

♦ In accordance with requirement of medical care practical applications, we'll continue to formulate and maintain common EMR standard formats for compliance by all hospitals and relevant industries and lay the foundation for inter-hospital exchange of EMR.

♦ Promotion of using EMR for hospital accreditation and health insurance professional examinations will relieve hospitals of the double burden of implementing EMR and simultaneously printing out paper medical records and effectively enhance hospitals' willingness for EMR implementation.

♦ We'll continue to research and discuss the ELSI issues pertaining to NHIP health information applications, review and replenish the required laws and draft the content and form for consent by stakeholders to guarantee public health information security and privacy.

♦ Provision of healthcare electronic certification service and electronic signature function will form a secure and reliable information exchange environment within the medical care system to ensure confidentiality, integrity, signer's identity identification and send/receive non-repudiation of medical care electronic data.

♦ Setup of public health information integrated application services will foster real-time, correct and accessible information to minimize duplicated data processing by the grassroots public health personnel, thereby provide the public the best public health services.

♦ Accomplishing setup of the health indices and fundamental database and completing the value-added application platform and virtual database will effectively manage the health index information and improve the operation efficiency and security of users in applying for health index information.

CHARNG-ER SHYU is a Counselor and Director of Health Informatics Center in the Department of Health, Executive Yuan, Taiwan, R.O.C. She holds a Ph.D. in Public Health and an EMBA degree in Information Management from the National Taiwan University. Dr. Shyu specializes in management of health informatics, biostatistics and public health administration. In 2002–2005, Dr. Shyu worked on the online health services initiative, utilizing Internet technology to develop various medical information operations, including patient data exchange, online transmission of medical images, and electronic certification of healthcare personnel and service providers. In 2003–2006, Dr. Shyu embarked on the online service project for local health departments, which entailed establishing health service portals and operational platforms, integrated planning and development of service systems and improving the information and network facilities of local health departments. Based on the outcome of her past projects, Dr. Shyu commenced the planning of National Health Informatics Project (NHIP) in 2006 with the goal of building an interoperable lifelong e-health information infrastructure. For many years, Dr. Shyu has been devoting herself to building Taiwan's health information infrastructure and the work of electronic medical record in the hope to create an environment conducive to the development of national health informatics and the nurturing of health information manpower.

ENDNOTES

1. http://www.doh.gov.tw/ufile/doc/.pdf

2. http://hca.nat.gov.tw/

Chapter 14

ICT in the National Health System in Spain– The Spanish Healthcare Model

Daniel Torres Mancera, Director National Observatory of Telecommunication and Information Society, Spain

Under the Spanish healthcare model all citizens have the right to health protection and healthcare service, as established by the Spanish Constitution of 1978. This model was specified under Law 14/1986, the General Healthcare Act, with the following features:

♦ Public finance.

♦ Universal access to healthcare services that are free of charge at the time of use.

♦ Political decentralisation of healthcare services to the autonomous regions.

♦ The provision of integrated healthcare, providing high quality levels, duly evaluated and controlled.

♦ The development of a new primary care model, with emphasis on the integration of personal attention and prevention, promotion and basic rehabilitation activities at primary care level.

♦ The integration of the various structures and public services dealing with healthcare within the National Health System (*Sistema Nacional de Salud*, SNS) and its organisation in healthcare areas.

Consequently, the National Health System is a co-ordinated ensemble comprising the central government's National Health Services and the Regional Health Services, which integrates all the healthcare functions and services for which the public authorities are responsible by law.

Law 16/2003, dated 28 May, on the cohesion and quality of the National Health System, establishes co-ordination and co-operation actions for healthcare public administrations as a means of guaranteeing citizens' rights to health protection, with the common purpose of assuring the National Health System's fairness, quality and social participation.

The central government's responsibilities in healthcare matters are to establish baselines and the general co-ordination of healthcare, foreign healthcare and international healthcare relations and agreements, as well as the legislation for pharmaceutical products. The responsibilities of the regional governments are related to healthcare planning, public health and management of the health services. Finally, local government entities are responsible for ensuring healthy living conditions and collaborating in the management of public services.

Due to the complexity of the Spanish healthcare model, in which the responsibilities and management of public healthcare services are distributed among different authorities, the incorporation of ICT represents an opportunity to improve efficiency and provide citizens with accessibility, security and streamlined response in any part of the country.

The National Health System Quality Plan[1]

In March 2006, the Ministry of Health and Consumer Affairs (*Ministerio de Sanidad y Consumo*, MSC) presented the National Health System Quality Plan, which contains six major action areas to address issues affecting the Spanish Healthcare System's main concepts and challenges.

The use of information technologies is included within these six major areas of action to improve services to citizens.

The growing use of information and communication technologies (ICT) is one of the key factors behind the transformation of healthcare services in the last few years. Today, ICT is present in both management and clinical processes, enabling the healthcare system to have more and better information about its own activities and results. ICT development, therefore, is a strategic factor for all the healthcare services and, consequently, for the entire society.

The use of ICT, both in Spanish and European healthcare, encourages the availability of online information and knowledge as well as coverage and mobility throughout the entire territory. Therefore, rollout of information technologies is at the heart of future highly transforming projects.

All the institutions have to make an effort to create a solid foundation that will enable healthcare information exchange between the autonomous regions, its extension to the National Health System and, in the future, to the whole of the European Union (EU).

The characteristics and complexity of the Spanish healthcare model where, in addition to the Ministry of Health and Consumer Affairs, there are seventeen regional governments involved, indicates that the experience in the rollout of ICT for clinical information exchange will be fully exportable and adaptable to the European environment, where there is also high geographic dispersion and a distributed healthcare system, the management of which is the responsibility of each of the Member States.

Over the last 15 years, the Administrations within the National Health System have been carrying out important initiatives to improve accessibility to and the use of its services. The regional health services have prioritised lines of action in the area of information technologies, taking into account a series of criteria that go from opportunity and feasibility to budgetary commitments. Despite certain diversity in the functional actions, all the autonomous regions coincide in three main lines of action.

The first of these is the creation of a reliable user identification system linked to the individual health card. The second is the development of the electronic health record for each user or patient within the area of responsibility of the autonomous region and the development of the National Health System electronic health record at the national level. The third major line seeks to provide an ICT-based system to enable rational and functional automation of all the processes required to dispense pharmaceuticals to patients.

The National Health System Quality Plan, therefore, embraces these common lines of action with a view to extending the benefits they provide within each region to the National Health System as a whole. To achieve this, it integrates the functional and technological elements necessary to make the regional systems interoperable throughout the entire country.

One of the strategies applied to develop these elements is the "Healthcare On-line" project, within the Avanza Plan, a government initiative that seeks to generalise the use of technology throughout Spanish society.

The Avanza Plan and the Healthcare Online Project

The Avanza Plan[2] was launched to respond to Spain's need to accelerate its integration in the Information Society, and its objectives are to increase productivity, strengthen the industrial ICT sector, encourage R&D and develop modern interoperable public services, based on the effective use of ICT.

The Plan is based on the European initiative "i2010: A European Information Society for growth and employment," presented by the European Commission on 31 May 2005, which identifies the main drivers for growth and employment as: knowledge, innovation and the construction of a fully integrated Information

Society based on the generalisation of ICT in public services, small and medium sized enterprises and homes.

One of the objectives of the Avanza Plan is to foster the use of ICT by public administrations to adapt their services to the digital era. The "Digital Public Services" strategic axis includes actions in the areas of education, civil registry offices, electronic administration and healthcare in order to achieve quality public services that are more streamlined, accessible and efficient.

Healthcare Online[3]

The Avanza Plan measures in the area of healthcare are encompassed within the Healthcare Online programme. The aim of the programme is to create the foundations for healthcare information exchange related to citizens and to take advantage of the potential offered by information technologies to rationalise processes, improve quality of services and to respond to the emerging needs of society. The programme seeks to encourage the use of ICT in the healthcare environment and so facilitate the work of healthcare personnel, improve services to citizens and stimulate clinical information accessibility through the creation of a healthcare intranet and a robust and secure central node, through which to connect the regional health services.

Interoperability, both in Spain and in the European Community, is a top level requirement. The challenge over the next few years will be to integrate the various solutions and platforms implemented by public administrations so that citizens can access the new services regardless of where they are.

The participants in this programme are the autonomous regions, through their Departments of Health, and the Institute of Health Management (IN-GESA), responsible for healthcare services in the autonomous cities of Ceuta and Melilla. The central government, promoter of the initiative, participates through the Ministry of Health and Consumers Affairs and Ministry of Industry, Tourism and Trade (*Ministerio de Industria, Turismo y Comercio*, MITYC), which has assigned the management of the programme to the public corporate entity red.es.

Objectives

The Healthcare Online Programme offers the health authorities a further instrument to fulfill their healthcare objectives, through the use of new technologies and joins forces with the autonomous regions and the Ministry of Health and Consumer Affairs in this sector in their quest to:

♦ Develop online healthcare services that improve the quality of citizens' lives and improve the efficiency of the health system.

♦ Complete the implementation of an interoperable health card system that will unequivocally identify the user throughout the entire National Health System.

♦ Deploy a central infrastructure enabling healthcare data exchange between the autonomous regions through a communications platform called "National Health System Central Node."

♦ Implement electronic prescriptions to reduce doctors' paperwork and unnecessary visits to the doctor, particularly by the chronically ill, and facilitate their access to pharmaceuticals.

♦ Enable electronic access to clinical data and progressively implement the electronic health record.

♦ Exchange digitised administrative and clinical information between the various regional health services in a streamlined and secure manner.

All this demonstrates the Spanish government's commitment to measures and initiatives that contribute to the implementation of digital public services in the area of healthcare.

Actions

The actions began in April 2006, with a total budget for the 2006–2008 period of €252 million, to which the Ministry of Industry, Tourism and Trade, through red.es, contributed €140 million, and the autonomous regions contributed €111 million.

In financial terms, the Healthcare Online Programme actions carried out during 2006–2007 represented 21% of the regional Health Departments' ICT budget for the same period.

Figure 1. *Total Budget (2006–2008).*

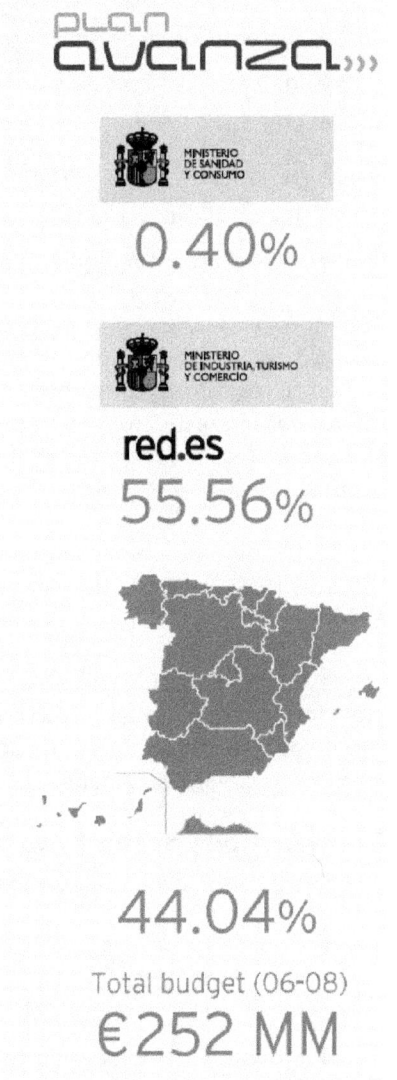

plan
auanza.»»

MINISTERIO
DE SANIDAD
Y CONSUMO

0.40%

MINISTERIO
DE INDUSTRIA, TURISMO
Y COMERCIO

red.es
55.56%

44.04%

Total budget (06-08)
€252 MM

Among the most important initiatives carried out within the programme are the following:

- The supply and installation of the infrastructure.
- Reinforcement of healthcare data processing centres.
- Enlargement of the National Health System central node, located in the Ministry of Health and Consumer Affairs.
- Development and implementation of the electronic prescription in two autonomous regions.
- Systems, services and/or processes integration projects.
- Infrastructure and network security.
- Storage.
- Support for medical image exchange.
- Telemedicine projects.
- Project co-ordination and management services.

The Ministry of Industry, Tourism and Trade, through red.es, acts at the National Health System level in co-ordination with the Ministry of Health and Consumer Affairs, reinforcing the central node in order to guarantee availability of the appropriate infrastructure for exchange of data associated to the new online services and, at the regional level, complementing the regional health services actions.

Project definition and specific actions have been carried out taking into account the situations existing in the different autonomous regions, their strategies and established plans.

These actions are being carried out within the National Health System's interoperability structural model, which enables interconnection of the various regional health services through the healthcare intranet operated by the Ministry of Health and Consumer Affairs.

Contributions of the Programme

The Healthcare Online programme is enabling:

- Consolidation of the commitment by the Ministry of Industry, Tourism and Trade to the development of public digital services and to the healthcare ICT sector, with an additional investment of €140 million.
- Provision of investment, technical advice and implementation capacity to the autonomous regions by the central government.

♦ Realisation of projects to meet the specific needs of each autonomous region and exchange of best practices within a broader National Health System agenda.

♦ Validation of a new management model in the National Health System in which the Ministry of Industry, Tourism and Trade, through red.es, has assumed the role of technological collaborator with the regional Healthcare Departments and the Ministry of Health and Consumer Affairs in the planning and implementation of ICT projects.

♦ Awareness raising regarding deadlines and key elements for carrying out information technology projects within the National Health System.

The period 2006–2008 has seen a marked acceleration in the actions that the healthcare authorities have been taking in the field of information technologies over more than a decade. However, the National Health System is facing important challenges that it will need to tackle in the next few years to complete the integration of the information systems in the National Health System as a whole. Progress has to be made in the integration of information recorded and stored in hospitals, and in the generalisation of clinical workstations in specialised services. Also, it is essential to consolidate the exchange of clinical data in some regions as well as to continue with the process design and definition of technical and semantic standards that will enable clinical information exchange and electronic prescriptions in the National Health System.

Currently, the integration of the various health information services associated with citizens (clinical information) is on the agendas of all the regional Health Departments, as is the exchange of specific data within the National Health System as a whole and, in the future, at a European level.

Results

Already, the first results of the actions carried out are beginning to be seen, although the degree of implementation in each autonomous region varies depending on the date of signature of the corresponding agreements and the nature of the projects.

The investment made has enabled the supply and installation of more than 76,000 ICT devices, as well as increasing storage capacity in various data processing centres.

To improve health services' equipment, over 60,300 PCs have already been installed in more than 6,200 healthcare centres, potentially improving services for 33.5 million people in these centres and for more than 253,000 healthcare personnel working in the different autonomous regions.

At the end of 2008, health cards in 15 autonomous regions had already been synchronised, and the two remaining regions had started tests to synchronise their health cards.

The capacity of the National Health System central node has been increased, creating a backup centre and an information security management system recently certified under the ISO 27001 standard by AENOR. The central node is ready to move forward with services such as the electronic prescription and the National Health System electronic health record, and to develop new clinical information exchange experiences between the autonomous regions.

All of this reflects the preliminary work carried out by the various organisations involved and the boost in investment and projects the Healthcare Online Programme is generating.

Behind these figures, there is a professional environment that is extremely receptive towards technology, highly qualified and strongly innovational, and in which R&D occupies a privileged place for developing solutions that can become international benchmarks.

The technological sector is taking full advantage of the opportunities presented by programmes, such as Healthcare Online, for advanced industrial development. This is enabling Spain, as a country, to develop a specialised industry that is already exporting specific ICT healthcare solutions all over the world.

All European countries are developing national and regional initiatives to enable healthcare professionals to access the clinical data of their patients at any time and from any place. In turn, the European Commission is co-financing the epSOS (Smart Open Services for European Patients) project as part of the European eHealth initiative. The aim is to create a European interoperability space that enables the exchange of clinical data and information on medical prescriptions between countries. Spain is participating with 12 other European Member States in the project through the Ministry of Health and Consumer Affairs and the autonomous regions of Andalusia, Catalonia and Castilla La-Mancha.

The ongoing actions are summarised below, indicating the agents directly involved in defining and carrying out the projects.

Electronic prescription in primary healthcare centres

Electronic prescription is an information system that enables automation of the identification, prescription, control and pharmaceutical dispensing processes (clinical cycle) as well as the administrative process for invoicing the prescriptions dispensed (administrative cycle).

It constitutes another step forward in the modernisation of the Health Services by incorporating benefits for citizens, particularly the chronically ill and their carers, reducing the pressure on healthcare personnel in the care provided by reducing the paperwork part of consultations, and giving greater streamlining and transparency to the administrative process, both for the public administrations and for the pharmacies.

The main objective of the electronic prescription is to free doctors from the administrative task of filling out prescriptions in those cases in which treatment continuity does not require review. Applying this philosophy means that a prescription is completed once, in a single action, for all the medicines that the doctor deems necessary and in the quantity necessary to comply with the indicated treatment guidelines and duration. The electronic prescription is very useful for the chronically ill and their carers, as well as to achieve rational use of medicines, improve treatment compliance, prevent the sale of pharmaceutical products without a prescription, prevent fraud and, in general, improve information on consumption and reinforce the role of pharmacists as healthcare agents.

Following the implementation of an electronic prescription system in a given health service, within the medium term citizens will be able to use this service in that region's pharmacies. In the long term, as the service extends to the different regions, this option will become available throughout the National Health System as a whole, regardless of where the prescription was issued.

In 2006, the electronic prescription had only been implemented in the health centres of Andalusia; the Balearic Islands, Catalonia, and the Basque Country

Figure 2. *Implementation status of the electronic prescription in health centres, 2006/2008.*

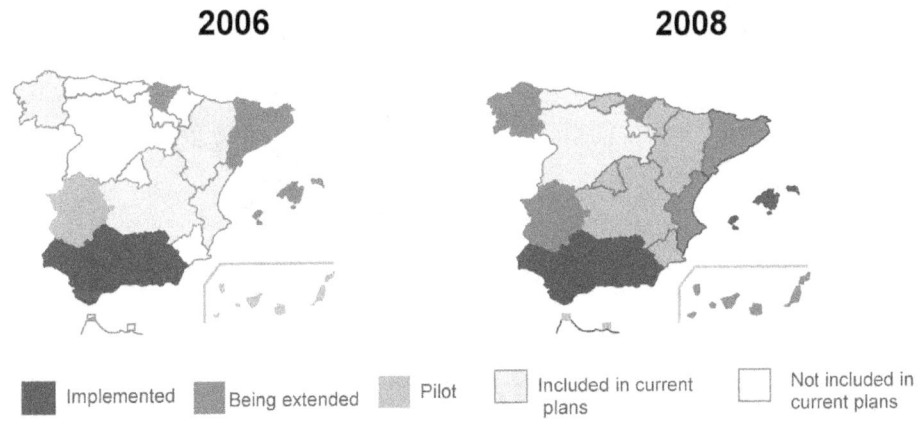

SOURCE: RED.ES

had taken the first steps towards the service, and the Canary Islands and Extremadura both had a pilot project. At the start of 2008, the remaining autonomous regions had already started, to a greater or lesser extent, to take the steps necessary to implement the service. There are now 5,500 paediatricians and family doctors with the service available, and 7 million citizens are attended at health centres that offer this service (the majority in Andalusia).

Electronic health record in primary healthcare centres

With regard to the electronic health record, the autonomous regions have been carrying out projects for more than a decade with the aim of setting up a single support medium to record the different contacts of citizens with the healthcare system (primary healthcare consultations, specialist consultations, hospitalisation, etc.) as well as diagnostic tests (laboratory, medical images, etc.), which would be accessible from any centre within the autonomous regions. The degree of maturity and development of these types of projects varies.

As regards implementation of the integrated electronic health record in the autonomous regions' health centres, in 2006, only the Balearic Islands and the Basque Country had implemented this service, though another eight regions were in the process of doing so.

In 2008, nine autonomous regions, as well as Ceuta and Melilla had completed implementation in their health centres, and another five autonomous regions were finalising their service extension. The remaining three autonomous regions were working on developments that would enable integration of electronic health records at this healthcare level.

Figure 3. *Implementation status of electronic health records integrated in primary healthcare centres, 2006/2008.*

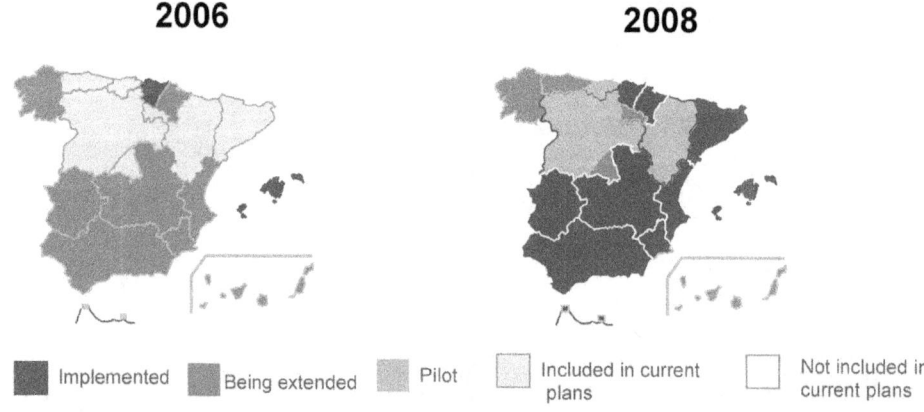

SOURCE: RED.ES

In the area of specialised healthcare, there is still much work to be done. All the autonomous regions have a high level of information and are working towards the integration of the various existing information systems in their hospitals. We can highlight the case of Galicia, where the Single Electronic Health Record (*Historia de Salud Electrónica Única*, IANUS) project has already been implemented in all hospitals, meaning that all the personnel of the Galician Health Service can access any patient's clinical and health information from any point within the Galician healthcare network, independently of where it was generated.

Online appointment system for primary healthcare centres via the Internet

In 2006, the health centres of the Canary Islands, Galicia and the Basque Country had implemented the Internet appointment system, and another four autonomous regions were about to do so; one had a pilot scheme, and four more were planning to implement it, as were Ceuta and Melilla, whilst the other five still had no plans to develop this service.

At the start of 2008, 64% of the National Health System health centres had the ability to arrange appointments with specialists by electronic means, and 21 million citizens have this service available to them. Catalonia and Andalusia have joined the group of autonomous regions with the service implemented, another five regions are in the process, and the remainder are planning to begin implementation in their health centres in the medium term.

Figure 4. *Implementation status of the Internet appointment health centres, 2006/2008.*

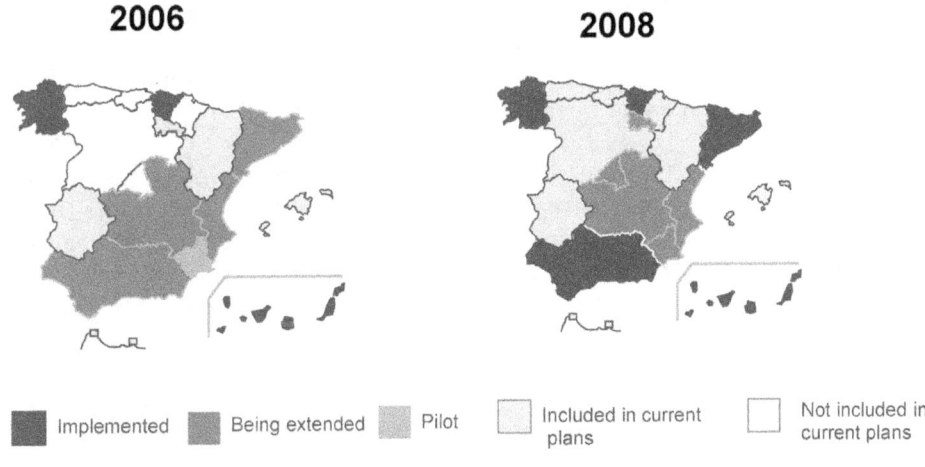

2006   2008

Implemented   Being extended   Pilot   Included in current plans   Not included in current plans

SOURCE: RED.ES

Conclusions

The use of ICT in healthcare and its integration in an overall healthcare model guarantees the development of a healthy society that is conscious of being properly cared for, enabling their mobility and ensuring coverage across the entire national territory.

The development of initiatives, such as the one being carried out within the Avanza Plan's strategic "Healthcare Online" project, guarantees the drive necessary to achieve results, such as the full interoperability of the health card between autonomous regions and the installation of infrastructure in more than 6,200 health centres, benefiting 33.5 million citizens and more than 253,000 staff.

Spain has achieved consensus on a model for clinical information exchange by means of a set of functional requirements agreed by all agents, enabling each autonomous region to have specific corporate information systems and for all of them to exchange data through a common infrastructure, the National Health System central node and the healthcare intranet. In this way, all levels of primary and specialist healthcare can interconnect, from small outpatient centres to large hospitals.

All the autonomous regions are developing innovative services, such as the online appointment system, the electronic health record and the electronic prescription, with the challenge being to complete their rollout throughout the entire regional territory. In parallel, the development and expansion of the National Health System central node enables the interconnection of the regional health systems, the interoperability of citizens' health cards and facilitates the retrieval and exchange of clinical data on a national scale.

The solution agreed for managing the interrelationship of 17 specific regional information systems for clinical information exchange has aroused the interest of other decentralised healthcare systems that have to integrate multiple information systems in order to offer quality services to their citizens.

Spain has, therefore, become a benchmark country at world level, and its healthcare model is being used as an example by other countries such as the USA. Spain is also in the lead in Europe in terms of the use of the Internet for training its general medical staff and above average in the EU in online appointments and communication with patients.[4]

Each day we find ourselves closer to the ideal of an Information Society in which staff and citizens have easy access to better and more structured information for making healthcare decisions, as well as access to better services, both at national and European level.

DANIEL TORRES MANCERA is a telecommunications engineer and has an Executive MBA from Instituto de Empresa and ISEM (University of Navarra). Since 2008, he is the director of the Spanish National Observatory for Telecommunications and the Information Society. From 2004 to 2008 he was an advisor to the Secretary of State for Telecommunications and the Information Society, and member of the board of directors of Inteco, S.A. (public company developing accessibility and e-confidence technologies). Prior to that, he was a strategic advisor to CEOs in the international ICT sector. He is a lecturer in marketing, finance and strategic development at business schools and academic forums. He has also worked as international co-operation projects director for the Spanish Human Rights Association. He has worked for 15 years on projects in Spain, Europe and Latin America in the areas of Information Society (eHealth, eEducation, eGovernment), business development, projects development, eBusiness and ICT and Human Capital. He has started up audio-visual and communications businesses and directed due-diligence processes for investment projects in multinational environments.

ENDNOTES

1. Plan de Calidad para el Sistema Nacional de Salud. Marzo 2006. Ministerio de Sanidad y Consumo

2. http://www.planavanza.es/

3. ICT in the National Health System. The Healthcare Online programme. Red.es. Ministerio de Industria, Turismo y Comercio. Ministerio de Sanidad y Consumo

4. Source: European Commission. Information Society and Media Directorate General.

Chapter 15

The Patient's Perspective– Empowerment or Bewilderment eHealth: Background, Today's Implementation and Future Trends

Alfredo Ronchi, Secretary of EC Medici Framework, Politecnico di milano, Italy

Foreword

How can we measure success in eHealth? Is it a mere question of money saving or it involves more? It is foreseeable a win-win strategy, better service, more success stories, less costs? Is eHealth an opportunity in order to bridge the healthcare gap around the world? What can we expect from virtual laboratories and electronic patient folders? Does online medical services impact on patient privacy? Last but not least electronic patient folders last forever as usually requested by law?

Moreover, very often we hear of user-centred design, interaction design and the positive effects that good "design" can have, especially for the industrial products and on line services, but what effect can exercise a proper design «indirectly» on the user? How much can do the "design" for our welfare, to help us feel better, in our home or even exert a positive influence on our overall health?

Healthcare sector cannot be considered as any other "eSector." What do patients, or more simply Citizens, expect accessing healthcare premises or services? What is really relevant for them in the different regions of the world (e.g. on line solution in order to check if a medicine is "original" or a dangerous clone)? Do the "big brother" effect due to remote monitoring and telemedicine[1] play a positive role in such a context?

What are the indicators of success of the operation, how do we determine the degree of satisfaction of the user? By "commercial" success, the content of dedicated interviews, the express appreciation?

The expectation of life in the last century has significantly grown up; if we consider this aspect as a performance indicator, we can probably agree on a positive trend. Performance measuring in the healthcare sector may be related to a set of parameters having as the main one the effect on the patient. Apart from this, we can consider organisational issues, time and money savings, information and knowledge sharing and more. Applications and services will cover information, monitoring, education, safety and more.

Recent background

The health sector, if compared with other industries in adopting information technology, suffered a delay of ten/fifteen years until recent times. Early deployment of health information technology (HIT as it was known at that time) was primarily for financial accounting of medical transactions. Even if in some way the health sector has been the birthplace of one of the most relevant and pervasive invention of the last century: the transistor. It was originally developed and patented as a device to fight deafness.[2]

Experiments with computerized medical recordkeeping began in 1960s mainly in the US. The first electronic health records (EHRs) was designed and deployed starting in late sixties and early seventies. By the mid of the seventies, approximately 90% of the hospitals in the US used computers for business functions, similar penetration in Europe. Hospitals use to access mainly big mainframes as shared computational resources in order to manage their own accounting systems. Later on, they extended the use to manage partial patient folders related to medical exams. In that period of time 174[3] sites in the U.S. processed electronic data with some medical content.

Major part of physicians adopted EHR systems in the 80s thanks to the diffusion on the market of the personal computer. Of course, PCs at that time they were mainly stand alone resources; few of them were connected to mainframes as "intelligent" terminals. The early use of EHR systems by medical doctors was mainly addressed to keep a personal record of patient references, specific health conditions and treatment and last, but not least, billing.

In the 80s and 90s, incredible steps forward in diagnosis and care were due to the increasing use of information technology, many times the re-use of computer graphics turned in medical imaging lead to cutting-edge medical systems. Moreover, late in the 90s the introduction of 3D colour graphics break the flat gray shaded and cryptic world of medical imaging. PACS (Picture archiving and communication system) and laser printers revolutionised the management of medical images as well.

In 1991, the Institute of Medicine[4] in the United States declared the computer-based patient record (CPR) as essential for health care, a message reinforced seven years later on the occasion of the revised version.

The idea to take advantage from facilities or competencies not available on site is dated some decades ago in the field of health. Tele-medicine, remote-ECG, tele-consultation and more are very well known keywords. Telecommunication networks and IT-enabled peer-to-peer connections and data transfer thanks to modems and, later on, digital lines.

For quite a long time, Healthcare Information Technology (HIT) has been mostly a chimera, and pioneers in the realm have faced relevant difficulties and unsuccessful stories. Some implementations played to role of bad ambassadors slowing down the progress. Some European telecom operators, for instance, invested time and resources in tele-medicine having no positive return of investment. Practitioners have generally regarded EHR as costly, cumbersome, and offering a little help for tasks at hand.

A number of experiences were carried out in the past, but these were mainly considered as experimental services. The incredible and quick diffusion of the Internet and broadband connection has to be considered as a turning point in the health care domain, as it happened in other domains such as eGovernment or eLearning. Internet and broadband enabled a completely new scenario: eHealth was born! The evolution trend was from *one to one* to *one to many* and *many to many,* and broadband made the difference.

Thanks to the characteristics of the Internet, some of the early projects addressed the need to exchange and share medical information more specifically the one related to rare pathologies. One of the first high-level projects in this field was the so called G7 CARDIO project (1993-95). The basic concept was to share as much as possible information and medical data related to rare heart pathologies trying to join the efforts in order to solve serious problems. Thanks to an innovative approach, multimedia documents such as medical standard pictures (DICOM) and medical standard video clips were available on line for the benefit of the medical service.

Tiny "computers" have been embedded in a number of portable medical devices and computer aided design systems become the digital companion of bio engineers together with nanotechnologies[5] and mecatronics.

The current environment in which health care is practiced and the information technology available to its practitioners are significantly different from that which existed in the last decades. Due to the Internet technology, the overall architecture of distance services has been reshaped, and a limited set of peer-to-peer services become, at the end, a full set of bidirectional multimedia interactive services including web 2.0 applications. There are differences in the temporal nature of information, the responsibilities of each member of the health care team, the need for a communications infrastructure to facilitate coordination of care, and other logistical[6] concerns which impact the detailed design of information systems.

Changes in the health care environment produced fundamental shifts in the delivery of health care, favouring outpatient care over impatient care, primary care over specialty care, and guidelines-driven care over autonomous decision making. Technological advances have overcome some barriers to computer-based patient records (CPRs) (e.g., World Wide Web, applications that operate across distances on many different computers) and heightened the visibility of others (e.g., confidentiality policies and legislation).

Let's try to better focus on this domain. A first attempt to classify the services might be by user: medical doctors, patient/citizens, institutions. Another potential taxonomy might be by service: web portals (hospitals, experts, medical/chemical companies, patients, etc), on-line or off-line medical care services (exams and consultation, virtual reality therapies, etc), management systems (medical unit information systems, etc.), and educational applications (medical doctors, paramedic, employees, patients and citizens). The opportunities offered by eHealth may benefit additional sectors such as rare pathologies, developing and emerging countries and "travellers."

From Medical Systems to eHealth

The rapid success of the Internet in the 90s reshaped the previous scenario based on peer-to-peer modem connections. At the beginning, already existent experimental procedures and trials were simply "rerouted" on the Internet. Very soon, experts found an incredible opportunity and completely new scenario thanks to the increasing set of Internet technologies. The very well known new opportunities offered by the World Wide Web drove a revolutionary vision that lead to the born of a new service sector: eHealth.

The term eHealth includes all the previous applications and technologies, but it means even additional services directly delivered to the citizens. One of the major characteristics of this new environment was the feeling of a more patient-centric concept of healthcare. The shift from technology serving medical doctors in caring patients to new technologies providing direct support to the patients had and still has a positive impact on citizens. Let us simply take into account unified booking centres and administration; thanks to multimodal access points (phone, Internet, SMS, etc) citizens may access medical services in a more rapid, efficient and even economic way. Healthcare institutions, on their own side, may benefit thanks to CRM, ERP, various database and optimization procedures.

If we consider as relevant in this field the trust relation between patients/citizens and the healthcare institution, a tight connection and timely personalized information flux from the institution to the citizen is surely one of the first step in order to achieve the goal. So far, SMS or email messages as a reminder for a visit, exam or simply providing operational instructions before any interaction with the Institution are probably appreciated.

The whole bureaucratic procedure related to exams, from the reservation phase to the delivery of the results if implemented on-line may save considerable amount of time and resources on both sides. From the patient perspective, this means less time devoted, no need to ask for one or more permission on the working place, no transportation fees, etc.

Moreover, the implementation of patient medical folders[7] accessible, with some limitations due to the privacy, on the Internet in a multi-language environment is usually considered an added-value service. Two main benefits are: the availability of the medical folder all over the world, good for travellers, and the opportunity to save and access the full set of information related to an exam (e.g. x-ray, CAT, MNR, etc).

Major part of such services is usually perceived positively by the citizens, there are of course some drawbacks in the implementation of similar applications. One of the first problems we face in implementing medical information systems is the lack of flexibility compared with handmade procedures. Additional troubles are caused by the rigid and traceable sequence of inputs and the enforced

Figure 1. *The implementation of the patient medical folder by ULSS 8 Asolo (Italy)*

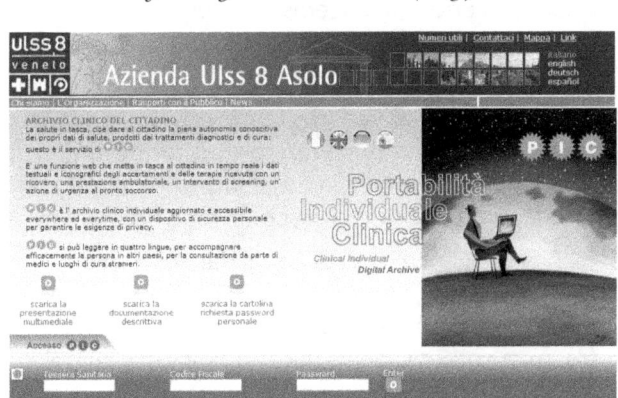

definition of responsibilities. Due to similar reasons is easier to start from "off line" medical folders, historical data then open folders.

The successful implementation of eHealth solutions including the deployment of interoperable electronic health record may, by principle, reduce the costs and improve the quality of medical care. Cost reduction may include:

♦ Innovative and better front office, including different communication channels (mobile phone, Internet, voice, etc), automatic resource optimization, automatic patient alerts, reminders and instruction;

♦ Improved and automated workflow both on the medical side and administrative side;

♦ Reduced expenses associated with record keeping (filing and retrieving paper based documents), easy document sharing among different offices and units;

♦ Reduced number of visits required, service delivery on the Internet (if possible—e.g. exam results, on line medical images, on line medical folders, etc.) including the availability of the full medical folder online in case of need even abroad.

Trying to summarize potential quality improvements:

♦ Real time information transfer and access thanks to intranet, extranet, and Internet;

♦ Availability and access, even from abroad, of a more complete and accurate set of medical data (patient folder) including documentation and medical images (e.g. CAT scans or X-ray images) usually discharged by the specialists because not strictly related to their specific needs (anyhow potentially relevant later on);

♦ Fewer dangerous medical mistakes resulting from poor handwriting or other order entry errors (this seems to be one of the most frequent cause of danger);

♦ Improved medical decisions through the use of structured data mining thanks to the creation of "ad hoc" ontology and specific tags. This enables to link together information related to the vast databank of historical medical folders providing and incredibly huge long-term knowledge base feeding health care decision support systems;

♦ Easier quality assurance and statistical data extraction.

This is simply a short list of both cost reduction opportunities and quality improvement tools, many other aspects may be pointed out in a longer description (social, cultural, etc).

The eHealth umbrella covers additional services including health care portals (medical units, drugs, care and treatments, rare pathologies and more) and the use of Web 2.0 features to support patient and citizens (e.g. patient blogs, rare illnesses portals, natural treatments,[8] etc.).

An example of online authenticity check of drugs is due to Sproxil.[9] Malaria kills over a million a year: a simple SMS could prevent 20% of those deaths. In order to fight the deadly consequences of the growing global counterfeit pharmaceutics market, Sproxil enables anyone in a developing country with access to a cell phone to authenticate their drugs before use. It works via a simple SMS, accessible by default on all phones, and available on all cellular networks. Akin to the very popular scratch card method for replenishing cellular talk-time, users reveal a single-use code on drugs and SMS it to a provisioned mobile short code, which, in turn, generates an automated verification response. There is no cost to the drug patron—genuine drug manufacturers are eager to bear the entire cost due to the entrenched benefits they stand to reap when counterfeiters are driven out of the market. Armed with a simple cell phone, users can finally rely on the quality of their medicine.

Another interesting on line service on drugs is Medicine Combination (http://medicinkombination.dk/). Medication can make one sick, if it is combined in the wrong way. Medicinkombination.dk helps multiple drug users to find out about how different drugs interact with each other. Users who take several kinds of drugs, herbal medicines, strong vitamins or mineral supplements can search on the website and quickly examine the consequences of their drug consumption and healthier combinations. The information on Medicinkombination.dk comes from the National Drug Interaction Database in Denmark which used by health professionals based on scientific articles and independent expert views. The user does not need to have any medical knowledge to use the service and a simple and straight forward interface makes the content service a perfect example for other countries.

As an example of patients active role on the Internet *Rate My Hospital* (http://www.ratemyhospital.ie/, see next page) is an interesting service. Have you ever been unhappy with a hospital? If yes, you will love Rate My Hospital! The web site is a rolling online survey of patient satisfaction with the Irish health system. In line with the best of social software sites, it provides a single, clear platform for feedback on hospital treatments and services. To date close to 10,000 people have completed a comprehensive 23-part online questionnaire on their experiences in Hospitals. The site aims to provide patient-centred transparency in the Irish Hospital system leading to improvements in the entire Health infrastructure.

Dealing with eHealth we cannot forget the eLearning services that may be delivered care of heath care institutions.[10] They may take advantage from the full

Figure 2. *Rate My Hospital web service (Ireland).*

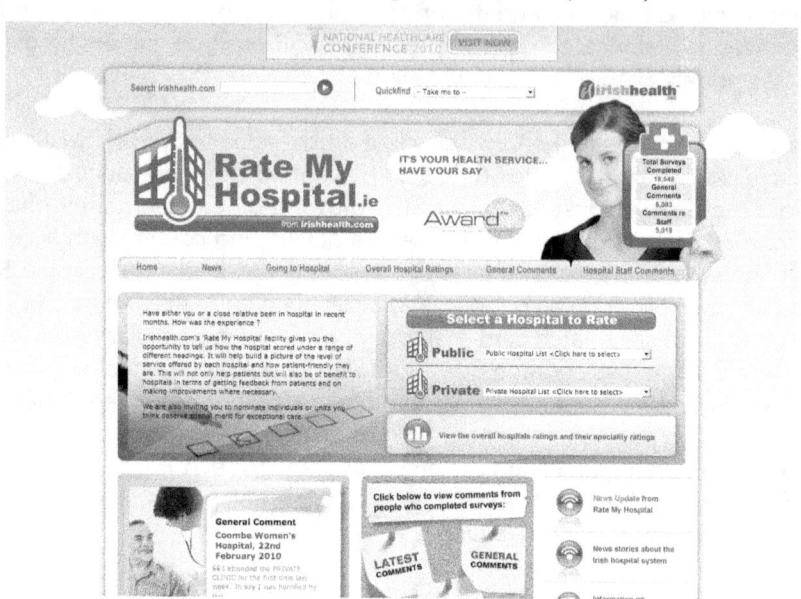

set of digital platform including podcasting and videophones and address the needs of a wide range of potential users from administrative personnel, paramedics, medical doctors, patients and even citizens (e.g. pandemic or first aid). Education and awareness are the goals of a set of application devoted to basic educational issues like sexual education and AIDS. Underworld (http://www.underworld.net.au/) is an example of such product. Funny, frank and funky sex education for teenagers: Underworld is an animated, interactive, musical, detective investigation into the female reproductive system. Part narrative, part documentary and a valuable source of information, the project explores issues of sexuality with humour, characters, songs and video. The CD-ROM includes interview footage with teenagers and adults, covering a range of topics including sexual preference, body image, young mothers, safe sex, first times and language. The detectives at Sam Sperm's Detective Agency are on a mission to find out what's going on during a menstrual cycle. And they also carry out other investigations.

eLearning projects and services devoted to young people do not cover the all sector. As it happens in other domains importance of Life Long Learning is growing and enlarging in every field: institutions, companies, governments and scientific communities recognize the importance and the need of continuous updating. Some countries made lifelong learning courses mandatory for medical doctors and paramedic personnel.[11] It is through interactive educational activities that the most effective learning is achieved. In order to improve the every-day clinical practice, it is necessary to develop new ideas, and this is exactly what experiential learning does.[12] Experiential learning is an outstanding breakthrough in the educational field and a new way to bring professional knowledge to the next level through a stimulating and memorable experience. Within the same domain we find, among the others, two relevant examples: serious games and virtual laboratories. Virtual laboratories offer, to a number of students and trainees the opportunity to put the "hands on" a laboratory trying experiments, making exams and more.

Both the use of remote labs and eHealth more in general may be the key factor in reducing the health care problems of third and emerging countries. As an example health care is one of the most fundamental needs for sub-Saharan Africa considering the region's multiple medical problems.[13] Tests are already been done and services on a regular basis are provided in different fields: tele-consultation, tele-diagnosis and even tele-surgery.

Technology also holds great potential for improving the quality of life of older people. For example, technology and telemedicine/e-health applications offer the possibility of increasing the physical and emotional well-being of older people and allowing them to remain at home longer.[14] With expansions in the 85 and older population, of whom approximately half require assistance with everyday activities, we will need information systems designed to help the aging to maintain their independence and meet their social, health, and other needs.

Technology can be used to monitor, from remote, people with chronic illnesses. This means to minimize the need to visit hospital's premises thanks to wearable medical equipments.[15]

Videoconferencing applications may also make it possible for physician to "visit" or counsel patients, particularly those with impaired mobility minimizing the need for travel. The Internet also affords patient access to a vast array of health-related information. It can also be used to facilitate communication between the patient and a provider, other family members, or people who have the same illness or disease (via online support groups and web 2.0 technology). Finally, reminder systems, such as automated messaging, can be used to remind patients of medications regimes, medical prescriptions before exams or medical appointments.

eHealth and privacy issues

Designing eHealth services, we must take adequately into account privacy issues. The healthcare sector is probably the only one characterized by a layered management of privacy, including limitations to the owner of the information him/her self. This is very often one of the major bottlenecks in healthcare service provision, the risk to infringe privacy rules and regulations.

As clearly anticipated by a number of movies, stolen digital identities, digital *desaparecidos*, and other digital crimes, these are the nightmares of the cyber age. Privacy is a luxury in the information age. In the near future, it will be necessary to find a satisfactory equilibrium between privacy and the "open" systems enabled by ICT. Security is one of the key issues in e-Health as well as a robust disaster recovery plan. Citizens must feel comfortable and in a trust relationship when they access and use e-Health services. The traditional trust relationship patient/physician has to be guaranteed even on e-Health platforms.

There are a number of regulations intended to improve health care data security. This is a side effect of the improvement of health care data access that has created new security risks along with headaches for patient and practitioners. If we refer, for instance, to the U.S., the Health Insurance and Portability Act (HIPAA[16]), enacted in 1996, have caused a major crunch for the computer security industry. "The Administrative Simplification provisions of the Health Insurance Portability and Accountability Act of 1996 (HIPAA, Title II) required the Department of Health and Human Services (HHS) to establish national standards for electronic health care transactions and national identifiers for providers, health plans, and employers. It also addressed the security and privacy of health data. As the industry adopts these standards for the efficiency and effectiveness of the nation's health care system will improve the use of electronic data interchange."[17]

Like many legislative initiatives, HIPAA appears to be intended to reduce costs, in this case insurance-related health transactions for patients, but as it happens frequently, the overhead of compliance has the opposite effect. Major part of potential information violations could be more likely to occur through electronic data collection and consolidation. We all know that privacy is an information age luxury, as much we use technology as much we are "visible." Privacy it is not costless. The privacy rule component implemented by HIPAA addresses the use and disclosure of Protected Health Information (PHI) by health care plans, medical providers, and clearinghouses. The aim of the Privacy Rule, accordingly with the U.S. Department of Health, is "The Privacy Rule applies to health plans, health care clearinghouses, and those health care providers who conduct electronically certain financial and administrative transactions that are subject to the transactions standards adopted by HHS.[18] The Privacy Rule requires covered entities to protect individuals' health records and other identifiable health information by requiring appropriate safeguards to protect privacy, and by setting limits and conditions on the uses and disclosures that may be made of such information. The Privacy Rule also gives individuals certain rights with respect to their health information."[19]

The key document related to the rule is the "Notice of Privacy Practices Patient Acknowledgement" form; we are already familiar with a number of it because of privacy issues in every field every time we transfer any personal data related with our identity. This form is usually one of the first documents we have to sign before receiving any medical attention from most health care providers. The usual purpose of this form is to attest that the patient (or guardian if a minor) has received proper information, usually printed in small on the same sheet of paper, regarding the use and disclosure of one's health care information (internally and externally the health service provider). The information may be provided to others beyond the medical practitioner's office. Estimates[20] in the U.S. indicate that as many as 150 to 400 individuals may have access to information collected in a patient's medical folder. On the contrary, giving the consent to the privacy form can mean that close family members may not be able to get copies of the contents or summaries of the medical records, even if this information is essential in order to obtain treatment or reimbursements. The same problems may be faced even in case of malpractice on similar medical cases.

Electronic patient folder: Is it forever?

In the previous paragraphs we outlined the increasing success and need of eHealth and specifically electronic patient records and digital patient medical folders. Apart from the basic problems related to loss of data or malfunction, there is a unique aspect related to medical folders: medical folders must be accessible forever. This is merely a question of conservation of physical archives all over the world if we deal with physical documents (documents, prints, images). On the contrary, if we have the right to turn physical archives into digital archives discharging physical originals, this is not possible without an explicit approval by authorities, we immediately face the problem of long-term preservation of digital documents.

People used to believe (and many still do) that digital formats were the ultimate formats for storing information indefinitely. The idea that texts, images and more in general data can be perpetuated by converting them into digital form is popular and widely supported.

As a result, a significant amount of our documents and data relies on digital technology. But is digital technology really suitable for long-term preservation? And are electronic devices, which are required in order to access information stored in digital formats, durable enough to guarantee future access to this information? If not, what can we do to overcome this problem?

The rapid evolution of technology makes the preservation of digital content a challenge. Considering the huge amount of data to be stored, including medical images due to NMRs, CAT scans, etc., the amount of time permitted to accomplish this task, and the length of time that such information needs to be stored[21], it is important to address the issue of the long-term conservation of digital information; a problem that has largely been underestimated up to now. Hospitals and health organisation are interested in the optimisation of physical archives; this sometimes means even reduction of the built surface devoted to host the archives. Digitisation seems to be an optimal approach, but the wise one suggests keeping the physical original in a safe "dead archive."

We need to consider two aspects: technological obsolescence and the temporary nature of "permanent" storage systems. Computer systems are aging; the media on which information is stored are disintegrating. Given this issue, what are the long-term implications of relying on current digital technology to preserve our archives?

Even if we simply focus, for the moment, on basic digital content such as text, we cannot guarantee that textual records stored in digital electronic form will always be accessible.

Storage media are subject to degradation; they are not designed to survive for long periods of time (the kinds of timescales associated with archives and governmental data). Magnetic technology does not guarantee long-term access to stored information; tapes and disks lose their properties and are sensitive to environmental conditions such as heat, humidity, magnetic fields, static electricity, dust, fire, etc.

In addition, they become obsolete as the devices capable of reading them become outdated and are mothballed. Old formats and standards are essentially shelved in favour of newer formats and standards.

This even happens for software standards, because ways of coding information and the quality of the information stored are constantly improving. This situation holds for both electronic records converted from already existent analogue forms (paper, medical images, video clips, etc.), and records that were originally created in electronic form (like it happens nowadays in medical imaging).

For digital content that is derived from an analogue source, the analogue source (provided it is still available—e.g. historical patient folders or temporary paper based folders) can be digitised again to new and improved standards and formats, so this issue is not a big problem. On the other hand, content that originated in digital form must be preserved based on the original record (e.g. digital imaging, digital signal streams, etc).

Until recently, documents were generally paper or film-based (X-ray, CAT scans and NMRs, etc.). Film technology was popular because of its efficiency, usability, robustness and we now recognise that it is almost hardware-independent. In the 80s the innovation due to PACS (Picture archiving and communication system) and its added value in managing medical images converted all the analogue images in digital images.

The life cycle of the data will influence its own creation and will generate an accounting record for the resources to be preserved. Since prevention is better than cure, if we define preservation strategies we are halfway to the solution. The preservation problem involves several other aspects in addition to the bare technological ones: there are administrative, procedural, organisational, legal, IPR and policy issues surrounding the long-term preservation of digital content. This increased complexity tends to be due to the different natures of digital and traditional physical documents. Online information such as web pages and databases are vulnerable as much as their web structure become complex thanks to hyperlinks and cross references.

At least one aspect should be investigated before settling on a particular preservation approach: the overall cost of preservation. This involves considering the best way to ensure future access to information during the design phase of the long-term data set. This approach may involve some feedbacks on the way to choose technology and standards and even the way to shape data sets. Once the data set is created, in addition to infrastructure costs, running costs may include: additional room on storage devices to archive copies and/or documentation and metadata, software applications that manage data refreshing, and costs related to porting or emulation.

A number of global studies[22] and projects have been and are being carried out into digital preservation; for instance the work carried out by the Taskforce on Archiving of Digital Information (94–96) on the mandate of The Commission on Preservation and Access and The Research Libraries Group Inc., as well as the OASIS Open Archival Information System project, CAMiLEON emulation and the VERS Victorian Electronic Record Strategy. Along with the ERA initiative launched by NARA, Interpares I, II and III are some of the most well-known projects in this field. In addition, a comprehensive vision of electronic record management is provided by the U.S. Department of Defence standard entitled the Design Criteria Standard for Electronic Records Management Software Applications (dod 5015.2 STD).

Finally, it is very important that research into digital preservation is carried out by strong interdisciplinary groups, since this should guarantee that an effective approach to a problem that concerns the foundations of the digital era is defined.

ALFREDO M. RONCHI serves as the secretary of the EC-MEDICI Framework of Cooperation, Secretary of the European Working Group on "EU Directives and Cultural Heritage" and head of the representative of OCCAM NGO at UNO International Centre in Vienna. He is appointed by ICNM as a member of Executive Board of Directors of the World Summit Award, member WSA Grand Jury and President of eContentAwardItaly the Italian pre-selection of the World Summit Award. He is member of the Europrix Top Talent Award Executive Board of Directors, programme Chair of different tracks and panels on the occasion of WWW, IEEE, Eurographics, Global Forum, Infopoverty and MEDICI international conferences and events. Alfredo M. Ronchi is appointed as eContent & Services expert c/o, the Norwegian Government, the European Commission, the Council of Europe, the Italian Association of Banks (ABI), National Research Council (CNR). He is member of the following scientific committees: Infopoverty, Fondazione Italiana Nuove Comunicazioni, Global Forum, Sacred World Foundation. He is a member of the Italian delegation for cultural heritage in the Italy China cooperation framework (2005-2009). Mr. Ronchi serves as professor at Politecnico di Milano (Engineering Faculty).

ENDNOTES

1. Term first coined in the 70s by Thomas Bird.

2. The invention of Transistors by John Bardeen, Walter Brattain, and William Shockley in 1947.

3. R.R. Henley and G. Widerhold, An analysis on automated ambulatory medical record systems, AARMS Study Group, UCSF, June 1975

4. Richard S. Dick, Elaine B. Steen, and Don E. Detmer, Editors— Institute of Medicine , The computer based electronic medical record: essential technology for healthcare, National Academy Press, Washington DC, 1991

5. Researchers working in medical nanorobotics are creating technologies that could lead to novel health-care applications, such as new ways of accessing areas of the human body that would otherwise be unreachable without invasive surgery.

6. In principle, in order to fully benefit from eHealth approach a general reshape of the organisation is needed including logistics and other infrastructure. Communication and access to information are strictly related to organisational and infrastructural issues.

7. E.g. ULSS 8 Asolo on line Medical folder https://servizi.ulssasolo.ven.it/Fpaweb/index.aspx

8. E.g. http://www.mamaherb.com/. Mamaherb.com is an internet platform, enabling users from all over the world to access and evaluate information on alternative remedies. Having become the world's largest free Natural Health resource, its goal is to function as a paradigm-changing tool in the field of alternative—and perhaps all—health related knowledge. Users are able to research, rate, comment on, or discuss particular treatments and thus, with the help of other assessment tools, such as links to external references, be part of a huge project which aims to assess the effectiveness of natural and alternative treatments. Exploiting the universality of the internet, Mamaherb.com seeks to address two main issues: "What's out there?" and "What actually works?"

9. Spoxil: http://sproxil.com/

10. E.g. the services provided care of the Medical Unit ULSS 8 Asolo, Italy—http://www.ulssasolo.ven.it/index.php/Area-informativa/Contenuti-multimediali/Formazione-ed-e-learning

11. E.g. ECM, continuing education programme for medical doctors in Italy—http://www.ministerosalute.it/ecm/ecm.jsp

12. A significant example of collaborative experiential learning is due to CELL (Centre for Experiential Learning) developed care of QBGROUP Padova Italy (http://www.qbcell.it/)

13. The World Health Organisation (WHO) reports that at the end of 2001, more than 70% of the people worldwide living with HIV were located in the sub Saharan Africa. Malaria is another relevant plague in the same area

14. A typical example in Europe is the Assisted Ambient Living (AAL) join programme. The AAL Joint Programme is a so-called "article 169 initiative" that was initiated by its member organisations. The status "article 169 initiative" was achieved only after the European Commission launched a co-decision procedure to which both, the European Parliament and the Council had to take a positive decision on the initiative.

15. E.g. wrist-watch like medical equipments able to track blood pressure, heats beats, skin humidity, acceleration, light exposure, etc.

16. http://www.cms.hhs.gov/

17. From the http://www.cms.hhs.gov/HIPAAGenInfo/ webpage

18. See 45 C.F.R. § 160.103 (definition of "covered entity").

19. U.S. Department of Health and Human Services, Office for civil rights. Summary of the HIPAA privacy rule.

20. Johns,M.I., HIPAA privacy and security: A practical course of action. Topics in health information management 22, 4 (May 2002) and Health Information Security and Privacy Collaboration Action and Implementation Manual http://healthit.hhs.gov/html/hispc/AIMReport.pdf

21. The time span is mainly related to the national regulations and data/ document type (usually forever).

22. E.g. The International Expert Meeting "Conservare il digitale", held in Asolo on 29 September 2006. The report, entitled Long-Term Digital Preservation: An International Focus (see http://www.ndk.cz/ dokumenty/asolo_memorandum.pdf/download), was created in order to provide some guidelines and suggestions on this topic— or http://www.digitalpreservationeurope.eu/

REFERENCES

Kirk L. Kroeker, Medical Nanobots, Communication of the ACM volume 52, number 10 September 2009

Brian Snow and Clinton Brooks, Privacy and Security, Communication of the ACM volume 52, number 9 August 2009

Don Monroe, Micromedicine to the Rescue, Communication of the ACM volume 52, number 8 June 2009

Medical image modelling tools and applications, Communications of the ACM volume 48, num 2 February 2005

Gladney, H.M., Principles for digital preservation, Communication of the ACM volume 49, number 2 February 2006

Bioinformatics: transforming biomedical research in medical care, Communication of the ACM, volume 47 number 11, November 2004

Sara J. Czaja, Starr Roxanne Hiltz, Digital aids for an aging society, Communication of the ACM, volume 48, number 10, October 2005

Peter G. Goldschmidt, HIT and MIS:implications of health information technology and medical information systems, Communication of the ACM, volume 48, number 10, October 2005

Victor W.A. Mbarika, Is telemedicine the panacea for sub-Saharan Africa's medical nightmare?, Communication of the ACM, volume 48, number 10, October 2005

G. Riva, F. Vatalaro, F. Davide & M. Alcañiz, Ambient Intelligence: The evolution of technology, communication and cognition towards the future of human-computer interaction, IOS Press 2005

David Merrill, Pattie Maes, Invisible Media: Attention-sensitive informational augmentation for physical objects, proceedings of The Seventh International Conference on Ubiquitous Computing. Tokyo, Japan 2005 http://ambient.media.mit.edu/assets/_pubs/dmerrill_maes_ubicomp2005.pdf

Alfredo M. Ronchi, et al,. Proceedings of the International Expert Meeting "Conservare il digitale," held in Asolo on 29 September 2006. (see http://www.ndk.cz/dokumenty/ asolo_memorandum.pdf/download)

Alfredo M. Ronchi et al., Design e Comunicazione per la Sanità (M. Maiocchi editor), ISBN 978-88-387-4321-5, Maggioli Editore 2008

ISTAG: "Scenarios for Ambient Intelligence in 2010—Final Report," IPTS, Seville, 2001

ISTAG, Strategic Orientations & Priorities for IST in FP6, ISTAG Report 2002

Mark Weiser's Ubiquitous Computing webpage: http://www.ubiq.com/hypertext/weiser/UbiHome.html

Mark Weiser's website homepage: http://www.ubiq.com/weiser/

Oracle Customer Relationship Management http://www.oracle.com/applications/customer-relationship-management.html

Chapter 16

Consumerism and Health 2.0

Jeremy Nelson, Afia Inc.

Personal health management has been one of the last areas to be touched by technology in a coordinated and automated manner. Currently, it is easier to find information about every credit card purchase and every bank transaction that you have performed than it is to get life-saving critical health information. There are many reasons for this lack of information, not the least of which is the demand from the people. To organize an individual's health information in 2009, one needs to get paper copies of every visit, every procedure, and every medication from every healthcare provider visited. The time has come for this to change, and the technology is now in place to make electronic personal health management a reality.

The true power in all of this arises from the process of giving people more information about themselves in order to make better-educated life decisions. The storage and retrieval of information has become so inexpensive that the barriers to providing this information are eroding daily. The Internet has created a platform to connect all of the disparate information about people's health into a single point that can be managed by the individual. In 2009, the U.S. health system is so fragmented and segregated that collecting the health information on paper for just one individual could be a full-time job. Consumerism and the future of healthcare can be revolutionized via three main areas: connected health systems, biometric devices, and individualized medicine.

Connected health systems

Tracking health information for an individual can be daunting in and of itself, but imagine the amount of information that a family has to keep track of. When you include the status of aging parents and extended family, the task becomes even more formidable. Most of this information is collected and shared in a colloquial fashion and is then, in turn, shared with medical professionals in that same fashion. It is quite amazing that the U.S. healthcare system relies on personal accounts to learn about familial diseases and issues that could dramatically impact the lives of the patients. There is a fundamental break down of information flow from patients to caregivers, and from caregiver to caregiver, that affects the overall health of the population.

Many problems contribute to the lack of information flow and accessibility in the U.S. healthcare system. For instance, in 2009 more than 50% of the physicians in the United States still record clinical information in paper records or in unstructured electronic data. The pure fact that the information is not even captured electronically makes it very difficult and time consuming to share. The process to get a copy of a medical chart involves one or more staff members performing the following tasks:

1. Receive the request for the record
2. Verify authorization to send this patient's information to the requestor
3. Locate the medical record
4. Review the record for what to send
5. Make copies of the record
6. Send the copies to the requestor

Simply having the information scanned into a document management system can save a tremendous amount of time, but then you need to decide what to scan. How far back into the historical records is necessary? Should we scan every document encountered moving forward?

There are still other hurdles and obstacles in place even if you have an electronic health record (EHR) at the physician's office or hospital. There are varying standards and formats to capture and transmit data. Many EHRs are not built in a manner that allows for easy communication with other EHRs and Health Information Exchanges. These EHRs were written and have evolved from a time when there was no incentive to share information and collaborate. The choice to upgrade or completely replace with a new platform can be very costly and time consuming.

Comprehensive health management is the holy grail of a connected consumer-powered health system, where patients and physicians are working together to manage lives and cure diseases. Chronic diseases such as cancer, diabetes, congestive heart failure, infectious disease, and mental illness are some of the most difficult to manage and are the costliest factors in the United States healthcare system. In 2005, chronic diseases accounted for more than 70% of all of the deaths and 75% of all the costs in the United States.[1] By creating tools and a platform for individuals to begin to manage their own health, we can truly reform healthcare. Providing tools to manage one's health won't necessarily guarantee that one will, but it will be a start, and a social effect can begin to take effect. This is true in the financial industry as well. There are many tools available, such as Quicken and mint.com, to manage one's own financial situation, but many people still don't. A whole new industry of wireless medical devices exist that range from scales or blood pressure monitors in your vehicle, to wearable materials that include monitors that can sense heart rate changes or a possible stroke and notify you or your healthcare provider before it is too late. One of the main reasons that people don't better manage their chronic health conditions is that it is often too laborious and time consuming to keep track of these things, and people don't want to think about the consequences. As we begin to create technology that will be less intrusive and gather information from activities and situations that people already engage in, then we will create an environment for change and improvement.

Figure 1. *Leading causes of death in the United States, 2005.*

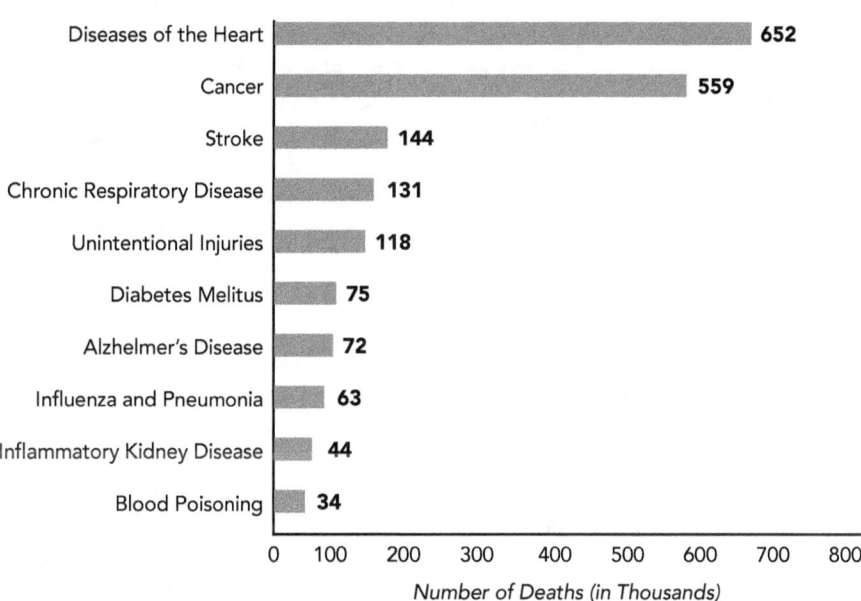

Number of Deaths (in Thousands)

SOURCE: Kung HC, Hoyert DL, Xu JQ, Murphy SL. Deaths: final data for 2005. National Vital Statistics Reports 2008;56(10). Available from: http://www.cdc.gov/nchs/data/nvsr/nvsr56/nvsr56_10.pdf Adobe PDF file [PDF-2.3MB] Wu SY, Green A. Projection of chronic illness prevalence and cost inflation. Santa Monica, CA: RAND Health; 2000.

Beginning in 2009, the United State federal government passed landmark legislation in the American Recovery and Reinvestment Act that laid the foundation to create a National Health Information Network that will incentivize physicians and hospitals to adopt EHRs and participate in Health Information Exchanges. All of this is important because it lays the groundwork to begin providing information to patients to help them manage their lives. Since the physicians have been historically responsible for maintaining the health records of individual patients, a lot of work is required to bring those physicians up to speed from a technology standpoint. As patients begin to receive electronic information about their health care, and tools are provided to help them manage that better, you will begin to see patients push physicians and require that they have systems in place to share and communicate about their care.

Biometric devices

As wireless devices are integrated more and more into centralized information tools for individuals, the promise of personal health management has great hope. Imagine that your cell phone could track all of your vital health information and provide real-time updates to your personal health record about your heart rate, blood pressure, caloric intake, exercise, stress level, etc. Wireless devices can provide location-based services, such as the closest physician location that provides a certain specialty, or what the best pharmacy or clinic is in your area that has an appointment available for you or your family. Continuous monitoring of health indicators can provide supplemental support for annual maintenance and check-ups to notify individuals of any abnormalities or changes that should be addressed quickly. Wireless devices will become extensions of us and will help keep track of key health indicators to assist in managing our care.

Social networks provide many great opportunities to influence and improve healthcare from both a population standpoint and a personal standpoint. Many of the health treatments and cures are shared amongst small groups of people in informal networks. Almost every person has heard a phrase similar to, "Well my friend had that problem, and she used ... to fix it." As we are seeing, there is great power in large communities of connected people working on complex problems and sharing information. Websites like patientslikeme.com offer people the ability to share their health story and collaborate on solutions and outcomes. This type of instantaneous information sharing allows for new possibilities in treatment and engagement that would not have been possible in the traditional doctor-to-patient interaction.

Social networks also allow connections at a virtual level that may never have been possible in a non-virtual setting. Many things—from personal exercise monitoring and competition, to online games that include health-monitoring statistics—can be created to provide augmented realities. The whole concept of interacting with and caring for elderly family that are in assisted living facilities could be completely transformed with virtual online games and video conferencing, along with the ability for family members to monitor key health information remotely. Some of this remote monitoring is already allowing physicians and healthcare providers to monitor patients in their own homes, which reduces the need to send them to assisted living and retirement homes. These types of enhancements improve the overall quality of life and don't replace the need for face-to-face human interaction, but can supplement the time when that is not possible.

Personal health information can begin to be monitored from a family point of view, and the family home can be used to help monitor and manage care. There are many things within the house that can be used to help improve health. Many new inventions can be created to use things like the bathroom mirrors to monitor skin changes, or kitchen appliances to monitor nutrition and diet. Families often have one person that takes on the responsibility of monitoring and managing the care of the individuals in the family. By having individual information accessible and devices within the home to assist, this job can be more easily shared and distributed. The possibilities are endless and can be used in ways to create helpful mechanisms to monitor health and improve care.

A large area for growth will be in nutrition and diet management with technological monitoring. There is already a large market for identifying and tracking what food you have consumed and calculating the associated calories. The iPhone and the Google phone have many applications that are already available and provide you that information wherever you are. The problem with the current information capture and monitoring systems are that they rely on the individual to remember what they ate and when and then remember to write it down or record it. This can be helpful and useful for people that are good at keeping track, but many Americans do not do a good job tracking or remembering that kind of information. There are many possibilities to start to make this process easier for individuals. Many foods that are purchased at restaurants or from fast food stores could have some sort of RFID or wireless transmission to an individual's wireless monitoring device that will indicate what was consumed and the caloric intake. There will be monitoring devices that sense the digestive system and can interpret and quantify the amount and what type of nutrients are being consumed and burned. The possibilities are endless, and it will take creative minds that can blend this sort of innovative tracking with what people would actually participate in.

Many efforts are already under way to begin to provide individuals access to their health information. Microsoft has created HealthVault, a secure online personal health record (PHR) where developers can create addons to link in their health devices and systems to the PHR. Google has created Google Health, a health platform that allows developers to create widgets to interface and interact with Google Health. Also, many individual insurance companies and physician practices have created their own PHRs for their members and patients. These efforts are still flawed in many ways because they require the individual patient to enter all of their own information, and then that information is not sent to or connected to their health providers. In many of the insurance PHRs, only your claim information is available, which can be helpful to see what procedures and medications you received, but they don't actually tell you anything about your health status or possible diseases. These are important steps in getting to the ultimate goal of fully connected personal health records for all citizens that can connect to all parts of the healthcare system that you interact with, and you as the patient can control how and where the information is transmitted.

Individualized medicine

Medications and pharmaceuticals have been one of the fastest growing components of the healthcare industry for the last two decades. There has been an explosion of new types of drugs for just about every possible ailment that exists; keeping track of which drug is for what or what all of the side effects and interactions is too much for one person. There are many databases out there already that pharmacies use that can warn people about possible interactions or side effects that they may encounter based on other medications they are taking or allergies they have. One such site is called epocrates. It is an online tool that allows both patients and physicians to search and learn more about what a medication does and what it looks like. Many older adults are on so many medications that they have difficulties keeping track of what all of the side effects are and what pills they are supposed to take when. This problem is reduced when there is another primary caregiver or partner in the house with the older adult, but imagine if they are living alone or in an assisted living facility. Wouldn't it be nice if that person could allow you to log into or remotely monitor their medications from your home? By having a personal health record where all of this information can be stored and processed, it makes it much easier to manage your medications and provide feedback on symptoms and side effects, so the next time you and the physician will be better informed.

As the U.S. population grows older, this problem will only increase and be exacerbated. Based on the 2005 MCBS study[2], over 92.7% of adults 65 years and older are taking prescribed medications, and that is up 5.6% from 1995. The data on children taking medications is astounding. According to a 2005 Slone Survey[3], over 54% of children take at least one medication weekly, and 20% take a prescription drug. The amount of information that individuals will have to manage and have access to will only increase, and technology will be the most efficient way to assist in the management of this data. Personal health records and health monitoring devices will be able to augment support and management for all people, helping them live healthier and safer lives.

There are some concerns that people's lives will be taken over and run by the technology and devices, but with the proper education and appropriate implementations, this technology can be additive to health and not controlling. Some medications also have many side effects that contribute to poor energy levels and weight gain, and PHRs can be linked with nutritional monitoring technology that helps combat some of these side effects and improve individuals' quality of life.

Personalized medicine will begin to transform the pharmaceutical industry as this information becomes more centralized and specific to each individual. Research in genetics is paving the way to become very specific about how medicines affect an individual's DNA and chemical makeup. Many medications are made for the masses and are tested on a cross section of human subjects, but each person has a specific chemical and physical makeup that may make certain medications ineffective or cause side effects that are undesirable. Personal health records and personal health management will begin to create a foundation for more real-time monitoring and a new breed of personalized medicine called pharmacogenomics that will be bring about unprecedented medical advances. Pharmacogenomics is the study of how an individual's genetic inheritance affects the body's response to drugs. This type of research and the possibilities of medical breakthrough will only be strengthened and enhanced with each person being able to participate and aid in their own health.

Many new employment opportunities will become available to assist individuals and physicians in the management of personal health information. Health assistants will be needed to help provide intermediary support and first-level health maintenance between patients and their physicians. These assistants could provide "Live Help" support inside of an individual's PHR, much like many websites have now for technical support. Each individual can ask for help and then allow that person to have access to specific information that is related the help request that they have. This could be part of a covered insurance service, or people could pay small fees to get the support. This would help save costs on going into the physician for an office visit and may assist the individual in diagnosing the severity of their illness. These types of intermediary support should help ease the workload of the physicians and reduce the wait times and amount of paperwork that patients experience.

Many other health assistant types of positions are possible, especially for specialties and hospital visits. There will be a virtual health navigator that assists patients throughout their visit and stay at a hospital. These new types of career opportunities will also require new types of educational requirements. Health assistants will have to be trained and certified to be able to provide the level of medical intervention that is needed, which will create new secondary education opportunities.

The future is filled with possibilities for all types of advancements and innovations in the field of personal health management. By empowering individuals with tools and support to manage their health, we will create a culture of wellness and personal responsibility that was only thought to be theoretical. The 2000s have brought many great achievements in both the medical field and personal information management. With electronic health records, personal health records, disease management systems, wireless health monitoring devices, and the Internet to connect everything, a foundation is being laid that will create a platform for a more engaged patient and a more informed physician. Individualized medicine combined with tools to manage the vast amount of health information that each person generates will allow people to make more informed decisions and enjoy lives that are healthier and longer than ever before. Personal health management and consumerism will revolutionize the healthcare system and truly give the power to individuals.

JEREMY NELSON is the Chief Executive Officer of Afia Inc., a health IT strategy and consulting firm based in Ann Arbor, Michigan. An expert on electronic health record design and implementation for behavioral and physical health, Nelson is well-known in the behavioral health IT field. He led the implementation of the award-winning Encompass Electronic Health Record (EHR) for five counties in Southeast Michigan as the Chief Information Architect at the Washtenaw Community Health Organization. He has been critical to the standardization of Health Information Technology in the state of Michigan as well as a key member of the SAMHSA workgroup team that developed the Behavioral Health HL7 profile.

ENDNOTES

1. Centers for Disease Control, http://www.cdc.gov/NCCdphp/ overview.htm

2. Medicare Current Beneficiary Survey, http://www.cms.hhs.gov/mcbs

3. Patterns of Medication Use in the United State 2005, Slone Epidemiology Center, Boston University, http://www.bu.edu/slone/ SloneSurvey/AnnualRpt/SloneSurveyWebReport2005.pdf